THE COMPLETE GUIDE TO HEALING FIBROMYALGIA

Deborah Mitchell

A Lynn Sonberg Book

St. Martin's Paperbacks

THE COMPLETE GUIDE TO HEALING FIBROMYALGIA

Copyright © 2011 by Lynn Sonberg Book Associates.

Cover photo by D. Hurst/Alamy.

All rights reserved.

For information address St. Martin's Press, 175 Fifth Avenue, New York, NY 10010.

EAN: 978-0-312-53418-9

Printed in the United States of America

St. Martin's Paperbacks edition / March 2011

St. Martin's Paperbacks are published by St. Martin's Press, 175 Fifth Avenue, New York, NY 10010.

10 9 8 7 6 5 4 3 2 1

CONTENTS

Chapter 4: Getting a Diagnosis

PART II: Take Charge of Your Life With Fibromyalgia

Chapter 5: Treating Fibromyalgia With Medication

Chapter 6: Exercise and Movement Therapies

Chapter 7: Alternative Mind/Body Therapies

Chapter 8: Herbal Remedies and Nutritional Supplements

INTRODUCTION

Millions of people in the United States and millions more around the world wake up each day feeling as if they had not slept and knowing that the pain they feel as they get out of bed will stay with them the rest of the day, and the day after that, and on and on.

They suffer from a medical condition called fibromyalgia. Some people with the condition will be too fatigued to make breakfast for their children or be in too much pain to lift their infants into a high chair. Young men and women in their career-building years may be unable to continue going to work and may face the likelihood of disability. Couples who once enjoyed socializing, going on vacations, playing with their children, and making love find that the chronic pain, joint stiffness, uncertainty of bowel problems, and overwhelming fatigue experienced by one of them has greatly stressed their relationship. Otherwise healthy-looking men and women who once jogged and swam and played tennis now find it an athletic event to walk to the end of their driveway.

Not so long ago, people who lived with these debilitating symptoms were told it was "all in their head," that they were imagining things, or even that they were crazy. If they could find a doctor who would listen and who was sympathetic, they might get a variety of drugs that did little or nothing to relieve their pain or the many other symptoms they were experiencing.

Thank goodness those days are over.

The good news is that the medical profession, the scientific community, and the pharmaceutical industry now recognize fibromyalgia as a legitimate condition. That means patients—most often women, because 80 percent of those with fibromyalgia are female—are much more successful at finding medical assistance; that research into the causes, prevention, and treatment of fibromyalgia is actively being pursued; and drug companies, seizing an opportunity, are developing prescription medications.

There is more good news. Although the symptoms of fibromyalgia are many and often serious, a growing number of people with the syndrome are finding effective ways to combat them. Some people turn to conventional approaches while others choose alternative and complementary therapies. This book offers you information and choices from both sides of the aisle and also discusses what many people with fibromyalgia are learning for themselves: combining conventional and complementary therapies is often the best way to fight this disease.

As Vera, a thirty-one-year-old fibromyalgia patient noted at a support group gathering, "When I first began researching all the different ways to treat fibromyalgia, I got anxious because I thought there were way too many choices. Then I realized that having many possibly effective options was a good thing. Imagine if there were only three or four treatments and none of them worked for me. Then what would I do? I actually feel empowered by having so many choices. I found what I call the three Ms that work for me: medication, massage, and MSM [a natural supplement]. Oh yes, and my support group, which is a huge help as well." Vera's story is not unusual: you, too, can find relief from fibromyalgia if you are willing to embrace the options available to you and find those that are most suited to your needs and lifestyle.

When compared with other health challenges that can be as debilitating as fibromyalgia is for so many people, our understanding of this syndrome is in its infancy. Diagnosis can be a very long process, often taking years from the time an individual reports symptoms to when a doctor finally identifies the syndrome. Once the syndrome is diagnosed, there are only three FDA-approved drugs specifically for fibromyalgia, although there are many other medications healthcare providers can prescribe for off-label use to treat the symptoms, and also many more natural and alternative and complementary options.

This book explores what we know about fibromyalgia and how individuals with the syndrome can live their lives to the fullest. In these pages you will find the most up-to-date information on diagnosis, including the new preliminary diagnostic guidelines (2010) from the American College of Rheumatology, as well as many treatment options from both the conventional and complementary realms, and suggestions on ways to improve quality of life.

HOW TO USE THIS BOOK

The book is divided into two main sections. The four chapters that make up Part 1 explore the syndrome of fibromyalgia: what it is and what it is not; a detailed evaluation of its signs and symptoms, and what they mean to people who live with fibromyalgia; how to find healthcare providers to help you get a diagnosis and treatment; and what the process of getting a diagnosis includes. These chapters help fibromyalgia patients understand the role they can play in getting a diagnosis and choosing treatment options.

Then in Part 2, "Take Charge of Your Life With Fibromyalgia," readers learn about all the options they have now that they have a diagnosis. The chapters in this section explore medications and other conventional treatments, natural supplements and herbal remedies, alternative/complementary therapies, different types of movement and exercise therapies, the role of diet in fighting fibromyalgia, the value of support systems and how to utilize them, and how to handle everyday activities and responsibilities when you have fibromyalgia, including what to do when you travel, how to restore your sex life, how to cope with motherhood, what to do about work and disability, and how to learn new sleep habits.

Having fibromyalgia changes lives—the lives of the people with the syndrome and those of their loved ones. This book is for all of you.

PART I

Fibromyalgia: The Syndrome

CHAPTER ONE

An Introduction to Fibromyalgia

"I wish I didn't feel so exhausted and in pain all the time."

"It's a struggle to even get out of bed in the morning. I have kids to take care of, but I can't even get it together to make breakfast half the time."

"I used to have a great job, and then I had to quit because the fatigue and the lack of concentration made it impossible for me to keep working."

"I don't know which is worse, the fatigue or the depression or the pain. All I know is, I'm sick and tired of feeling sick and tired."

Do any of these statements describe you? If so, you may be one of the millions of people in the United States who is living with fibromyalgia. We say "millions" because it is difficult to obtain an accurate number of people who have fibromyalgia. Depending on the source, the numbers range from 6 to 12 million. According to the Mayo Clinic, for example, 2 percent of the American population has the syndrome, which places the figure at around 6 million. The National Fibromyalgia Association estimates the number to be 10 million in the United States and that this syndrome affects 3 to 6 percent of the world's population. If you check with WebMD, a popular Web site among Internet surfers looking for health-related information, you will see the high figure of 12 million Americans.

Why is there such a large range in estimates? One reason is that fibromyalgia is difficult to diagnose; another is that it can take several years of going to doctors before an individual is finally given a diagnosis. Many cases are believed to go unreported or undocumented because some people just give up seeking a medical reason for their symptoms. Quite simply, they are sick and tired of being sick and tired, and that no one can seem to tell them why.

Then there is the controversy among some physicians: does fibromyalgia really exist? It would be hard to convince the millions of people who have it that it does not, and indeed there is plenty of evidence that it does exist. However, a few physicians still shake their heads whenever the topic comes up. On January 14, 2008, *The New York Times* had a front-page story entitled "Drug approved. Is disease real?" with the subtitle, "Some doctors dispute existence of pain." The drug referred to was pregabalin (Lyrica), the first prescription medication approved by the Food and Drug Administration (FDA) for treatment of fibromyalgia—the "nonexistent" disease. (Actually, fibromyalgia is a syndrome and not a disease, but we explain that below.)

Although fibromyalgia is admittedly a challenge to diagnose and to treat, it is also a challenge to live with. We want to assist you in taking on these challenges and help you manage your "relationship" with this syndrome and with yourself.

So do not worry about the numbers: the number you should be concerned with is one, whether it is you or a loved one who has fibromyalgia or who is displaying symptoms. Regardless of how many millions of people are affected by fibromyalgia, the important thing for you to do is to gather all the information you can and seek help. And there's no better time to begin than right now.

WHAT IS FIBROMYALGIA?

The word "fibromyalgia" comes from "fibro," referring to fibrous tissue such as ligaments and tendons; "my" which refers to muscles; and "algia," which means pain. Fibromyalgia is a common, chronic pain disorder that impacts an individual on every level: physical, mental, emotional, social, and spiritual. Along with the persistent pain, individuals with fibromyalgia experience fatigue that can often be overwhelming, and a multitude of other physical and psychological symptoms that can affect all the organ systems in the body.

Fibromyalgia is a syndrome, not a disease. A disease is defined as a medical condition for which there is a particular cause or causes and signs and symptoms that can be recognized. This differs from a syndrome, which is a collection of signs, symptoms, and medical problems that occur together but are not related to one specific, identifiable cause.

Fibromyalgia is generally accepted as a type of arthritis, but unlike most forms of arthritis, fibromyalgia primarily affects the muscles rather than the joints. Although fibromyalgia is a chronic condition, there are a few promising facts we can say about it. One, it is not a fatal condition, and the pain generally does not worsen over time. Two, remission can occur when individuals participate in therapy and healthful lifestyle choices.

Among all the challenges that fibromyalgia patients face, there is also the frustration factor. Few people understand the condition, and it can be very difficult for family members and friends to relate to what an individual with fibromyalgia experiences every day of her or his life. If you are a mother who has fibromyalgia, you may hear "Why is mommy so tired all the time?" Your symptoms may have caused you to quit your job, stop seeing friends or entertaining, and cancel travel plans. Sexual intimacy may seem impossible. You may be too tired or depressed or uncomfortable to care much about anything except wanting to feel better.

The second part of this book goes into detail about how you can manage your symptoms and deal with the emotional and social challenges of this syndrome. For now, let's take a closer look at the syndrome itself.

WHO GETS FIBROMYALGIA?

Fibromyalgia is typically thought of as a woman's disease. Indeed, research indicates that 70 to 90 percent of those affected by the syndrome are females, and that the diagnosis is usually made between the childbearing ages of 20 and 50. However, according to the American College of Rheumatology's classification of fibromyalgia, about 8 percent of adults have the syndrome by age 80. Fibromyalgia is often seen in families, among siblings or mothers and their children. Men are also affected by the syndrome, as are children.

Men and Fibromyalgia

"How did I get a woman's disease?" That is a common question among the men who are diagnosed with fibromyalgia. In fact, men often have a difficult time getting diagnosed properly—more so than women do. As a result, it is believed many men with fibromyalgia are undiagnosed and so their cases are unreported. This has led some experts to suggest that the number of men suffering from the syndrome could be closer to 30 percent of all sufferers.

Men and women may not experience fibromyalgia in the same way. Symptoms in men tend to be milder, and men also reportedly experience fewer of the common symptoms, including fatigue, morning stiffness, and irritable bowel syndrome. At least one study, however, reported that symptoms in men were actually more severe than those experienced by women.

It is difficult to get a clear picture of how fibromyalgia affects men for several reasons: the condition is largely viewed as a woman's disease and so some doctors do not believe that men can get the syndrome; men are often reluctant to admit to severe pain or discomfort and so don't seek help; and men generally are expected to bear pain quietly and so do not seek active treatment for fibromyalgia even if they do get diagnosed.

Fibromyalgia in Children

It is estimated that one in six people who suffers with fibromyalgia is younger than 18. The encouraging news about childhood fibromyalgia is that children who develop the syndrome tend to have a better diagnosis than adults. Several studies report that more than 50 percent of children with fibromyalgia recover within two to three years of experiencing symptoms.

As in adults, among children fibromyalgia affects females more than males, and diagnosis is a challenge because the symptoms are often mistaken for those of other disorders and diseases. Fibromyalgia can have a major impact on a child's health and quality of life, because the symptoms can make it difficult for him or her to attend school, play with friends, and participate in routine childhood activities. Children who have a parent with fibromyalgia are more likely to develop the condition, as fibromyalgia has a genetic component. (In Chapter 10, see "Raising a Child Who Has Fibromyalgia.")

WHAT CAUSES FIBROMYALGIA?

This is a question that researchers would love to answer with confidence, but so far all they have are theories. For one thing, thus far no tests or physical examinations have indicated any major cause of the syndrome. For another, it affects a wide range of people: young, middle-aged, seniors, children, women, and men. Finding a clue to the cause of fibromyalgia among this immense population is a monumental task, but it is one that scientists are aggressively pursuing.

The Misfire Theory

The theory that has drawn a great deal of attention is that the brain's autonomic nervous system, which controls various bodily processes such as digestion, metabolism, and re-action to stress, misfires. Many researchers are focusing on the idea that problems with the neurotransmitters (chemicals in the brain that allow nerve cells to communicate with each other) and hormones used by the autonomic nervous system can cause certain bodily functions to malfunction, resulting in fibromyalgia symptoms.

For example, investigators have found elevated levels of a neurotransmitter called substance P in the spinal cord of patients with fibromyalgia. Substance P works as a pain mes-senger, and high levels of this neurotransmitter can cause pain messages to be sent to the brain even when there is no injury or illness that might cause pain.

Another neurotransmitter called serotonin exists in very low levels in fibromyalgia patients. Low levels of this chemical may explain why fibromyalgia patients experience chronic pain. Yet another neurotransmitter, tryptophan, is associated with sleep. Do you know why many people fall asleep easily after eating turkey on Thanksgiving? Because turkey contains high amounts of tryptophan, a chemical that promotes sleep. In people who have fibromyalgia, levels of this neurotransmitter are deficient, and this may explain why so many people with the syndrome have sleep difficulties.

The fact that fibromyalgia primarily strikes women most often suggests that hormones play a role in the syndrome.

Symptoms of fibromyalgia tend to be more severe in women who have gone through menopause, and the syndrome often begins between the middle to late forties in women, which is around the time estrogen levels begin to decline and menopause is on the horizon. Coincidence? Researchers are exploring this possible cause as well.

Excess Phosphate Theory

An endocrinologist and assistant clinical professor at the University of California, Dr. R. Paul St. Amand, was one of the first scientists to suggest that excess phosphate is the cause of fibromyalgia. In fact, Dr. St. Amand developed an entire treatment regimen based on this theory, in which he uses low doses of a drug called guaifenesin to alleviate

DID YOU KNOW?

Scientists have been able to "see" fibromyalgia using single photon emission computed tomography (SPECT). In a study of 20 women diagnosed with fibromyalgia and 10 healthy women as a control group, researchers used SPECT and confirmed that the women with the syndrome showed brain perfusion (the amount of blood flowing through the brain) abnormalities in comparison with healthy volunteers. These abnormalities were directly correlated to the severity of the syndrome, and the perfusion abnormalities were discovered in the area of the brain known to discriminate pain intensity. In addition, a decrease in perfusion was seen in areas thought to be involved in emotional responses to pain.

fibromyalgia pain and muscle tension. We discuss this treatment approach in Chapter 5.

Other Theories

Another theory involves the role of sleep. The majority of people with fibromyalgia have difficulty sleeping, and some experts suggest that rather than sleep problems being a symptom, perhaps they are a cause. The suggestion is that because fibromyalgia patients cannot get enough sleep, the body is not able to repair its injured muscles and nerves, resulting in serious pain.

The trauma theory is another idea. Many people with fibromyalgia have suffered serious injury or muscle trauma, often from an automobile accident, before the onset of their symptoms. Injury to the central nervous system can have an impact on how the brain functions and increase a person's sensitivity to pain, disturb their sleep patterns, and disrupt their cognitive thought processes. Thus, some scientists believe in the trauma/injury theory to explain fibromyalgia.

Infections that attack the central nervous system and inhibit the production of neurotransmitters is another possible cause. It is also possible for infections to cause damage to muscles, which can develop into chronic and widespread pain. Some experts suggest that fibromyalgia is the result of an overactive immune system: because it works so hard to protect the body against invading agents, severe inflammation and pain develop.

RISK FACTORS

There is often a fine line between a risk factor and a cause of a condition, and this is also true for fibromyalgia. However, we have separated out what are generally regarded as risk factors.

DID YOU KNOW?

In October 2009, preliminary research linked chronic fatigue syndrome to a retrovirus called XMRV, and according to unpublished data, possibly fibromyalgia as well. Scientists at Whittemore Peterson Institute discovered a retrovirus in the majority of chronic fatigue patients. When they tested some blood samples from people with fibromyalgia, they found a high prevalence in those samples as well. However, very little additional information is available at this time, and further research is needed to determine if there is a link between the retrovirus and fibromyalgia.

- **Age.** Fibromyalgia tends to develop during early and middle adulthood, but as we have already noted, it can also occur in children and in older adults.

- **Sex.** Females are more likely to develop fibromyalgia than males.

- **Genetics/family history.** You are more likely to develop fibromyalgia if you have a relative who also has the syndrome. One study found that 28 percent of the children of mothers with fibromyalgia also developed the syndrome. Another study reported that 66 percent of parents of children with fibromyalgia had some kind of chronic pain, and about 10 percent had fibromyalgia.

- **Overweight/obesity.** New research published in the May 2010 issue of *Arthritis Care & Research* reports that overweight and obese women, especially those who get one hour or less of exercise per week, are at higher risk for developing fibromyalgia.

• **Rheumatic disease.** People who have a rheumatic disease, such as rheumatoid arthritis, lupus, or ankylosing spondylitis may be more likely to develop fibromyalgia.

THE BOTTOM LINE

Fibromyalgia is a complex syndrome, and its causes are complex as well. Knowing what causes this syndrome would certainly help healthcare professionals develop more effective and sophisticated treatment plans. Until then, there are many options you can explore, as we discuss in the chapters that follow.

CHAPTER TWO

Signs and Symptoms

The signs and symptoms of fibromyalgia are funny. No, not "ha ha" funny, but funny in that they can appear and fluctuate in severity depending on numerous factors, such as weather conditions, stress, level of physical activity, poor nutrition, hormone fluctuations, and the time of day. These and other variables, when combined with the many different symptoms that can affect a person who has fibromyalgia, add to the complexity of the syndrome. As one forty-seven-year-old woman who had been diagnosed with fibromyalgia three years previously noted, "my symptoms are all over the map. And the journey is wearing me out."

According to Andrew Weil, MD, founder and director of the Arizona Center for Integrative Medicine, fibromyalgia symptoms usually develop gradually in people in their twenties, and the symptoms may fluctuate, flaring up and subsiding over different spans of time. Let's look at the symptoms together and see if what you learn about them can help you better manage them.

PAIN

The one overriding symptom associated with fibromyalgia is widespread chronic muscle pain, usually described as

SYMPTOMS OF FIBROMYALGIA

Muscle pain (persistent)
Fatigue (extreme exhaustion)
Joint pain
Sleep disturbances
Headache
Irritable bowel syndrome
Fibrofog (difficulty concentrating)
Confusion, impaired attention
Hypersensitivity to chemicals, allergens
Hypersensitivity to alcohol, medications
Mood swings, depression
Anxiety
Numbness or tingling sensations
Painful menstrual periods
Shortness of breath
Carpal tunnel syndrome-like pains
Vision problems
Sensitivity to temperature changes
Constipation or diarrhea
Nausea, indigestion
Dizziness
Low blood pressure
Heart palpitations
Frequent infections
Weight changes—gain or loss

dull, aching, stabbing, burning, or any combination of these. Pain and accompanying stiffness is often worse in the morning when you first wake up. The American College of Rheumatology established diagnostic guidelines for fibromyalgia in 1990, which spell out the characteristics of the pain necessary for an "official" diagnosis of the syndrome. These criteria are guidelines only, as some physicians do not agree with them: some say they are too strict while others say they do not go far enough.

Then in May 2010, the American College of Rheumatology published a new set of criteria for fibromyalgia in its journal, *Arthritis Care & Research*. According to Erin Latimer, Director of Public Relations at the American College of Rheumatology, the new criteria are preliminary, which means physicians can choose to use them or to refer to the original criteria when evaluating patients. The preliminary guidelines will not be made "official criteria" until they have been tested by an unbiased research team.

Essentially, the preliminary criteria replace the tender point test with a widespread pain index and a symptom severity scale. We cover the details of these two sets of guidelines in Chapter 4 when we discuss diagnosing fibromyalgia. What are "tender points"? We're glad you asked, so we will explain them right now, because knowing what they are will help you better understand the pain you are experiencing. Also chances are your doctor will look for tender points whether or not he or she uses them as the official diagnostic criteria, which we cover in Chapter 4.

What Are Tender Points?

Tender points, also called trigger points, are areas of tenderness around joints, but not the actual joints themselves. As stated in the American Rheumatology Association guidelines, these tender points hurt when they are pressed with a finger or a special instrument your doctor may use called a doximeter or dolorimeter. Tender points are about the size of a dime, and when pressed they typically cause a person with fibromyalgia to flinch or pull away, while pressing around the tender point rather than directly on it does not cause the same reaction.

Tender points are *not* acupuncture or acupressure points, but experts do not know what causes these localized areas of pain. So far they do not appear to be associated with inflammation, and researchers know that the location of these tender points is very specific, not random. This is helpful because it means that people with fibromyalgia experience similar symptoms associated with these trigger points.

Although the presence of tender points is a good indication of the presence of fibromyalgia and can help your doctor with his or her diagnosis, it is not definitive evidence. You should also tell your doctor about any other pain and all other symptoms you experience so he or she can use the information to help with a diagnosis. (See Chapter 4 on getting a diagnosis.)

More About Fibromyalgia Pain

Fibromyalgia pain affects the skeletal muscles, tendons, and ligaments, and it may cause your muscles to feel like they have been pulled or strained even if you have not exercised. Your muscles may twitch uncontrollably, and you may experience achiness around your joints. You may also feel pain in the bursa, which are the sacs that surround the joints, providing them with nourishment and lubrication so you can move.

People with fibromyalgia have a lower threshold for pain than people who do not have the syndrome. Experts believe one explanation is that the transmission of pain signals in the central nervous system is disrupted in some way so that fibromyalgia patients process pain signals differently than people without the condition. The National Institute of Arthritis and Musculoskeletal and Skin Diseases has conducted research in which they show that people with fibromyalgia have reduced blood flow to areas of the brain that help the body cope with pain. People with fibromyalgia also tend to be overly sensitive to touch, experiencing pain from stimuli that is not painful to other people. This is known as hyper-algesia.

Chronic pain is pain that lasts much longer than you would expect it to last based on the original injury or problem. With fibromyalgia, the cause of the pain is unknown, yet the pain persists. Chronic pain takes a toll on the body and is associated with abnormalities in brain hormone levels, low energy, mood disorders, muscle pain, and problems with mental performance. Neurochemical changes in your body increase your sensitivity to pain, which in turn makes chronic pain worse. As the chronic pain gets worse, you begin to experience pain in other parts of your body that do not normally hurt, and the pain becomes widespread.

Head Pain

One of those "other" areas of pain is in the head. About 50 percent of fibromyalgia patients experience chronic headaches. The National Fibromyalgia Research Foundation notes that most head pain that affects fibromyalgia patients is either a tension headache or a migraine. Some people have temporomandibular joint (TMJ) problems that can cause head pain, jaw pain, and dizziness, or head pain may have originated from tender points in the neck and shoulder areas. Other possible causes may include hormonal changes in women, dry eye syndrome, and side effects from medications used to treat fibromyalgia, such as tricyclic antidepressants, beta-blockers, migraine medications, and muscle relaxants.

Because the type of headaches may vary from day to day, it can be helpful to write down each headache episode and note where the pain is, any events or circumstances that may have precipitated it, how long it lasts, and if you take any medications to treat it. This information may help your doctor decide which course of medical or alternative treatment is needed.

Myofascial Pain Syndrome

About half of people who have fibromyalgia also suffer from myofascial pain syndrome, which is another form of chronic pain that can impact the entire body, but especially the jaw and face. At one time, researchers believed that myofascial pain syndrome was a type of fibromyalgia, but they now know that they are separate conditions.

Myofascial syndrome affects the muscles and fascia throughout the body. Fascia is like a web of connective tissue that surrounds the bones, tissues, organs, and blood vessels. This syndrome can attack the fascia and cause it to break down, resulting in chronic pain that can be stabbing, aching, throbbing, and when severe, debilitating.

The pain associated with myofascial syndrome originates in specific sites on the body, called myofascial trigger points. These points, unlike fibromyalgia tender points, feel like tiny bumps or nodules under the skin. Myofascial trigger points develop where the fascia makes contact with a muscle. When myofascial trigger points are pressed, they produce pain and muscle twitching. In many cases, the pain is felt in an area distant from the spot that you or your doctor press. This is called *referred pain*.

Pain associated with myofascial syndrome is often located in the jaw, although any part of the body can be affected. Myofascial pain can also produce other symptoms, some of which are also associated with fibromyalgia. These include:

• Numbness in the extremities

• Popping or clicking of the joints

• Limited movement of the joints, especially the jaw

• Migraine or headache

- Sleep disturbances

- Balance problems

- Muscle weakness (e.g., dropping things)

- Memory problems

- Ringing in the ears or ear pain

- Double or blurry vision

- Unexplained nausea, dizziness, and sweating

These symptoms can be made worse by factors such as stress, weather changes (sudden cold, high humidity, extreme dryness), and physical activity. In this way, myofascial pain is similar to fibromyalgia.

It is important that your doctor be able to distinguish myofascial pain from pain associated with fibromyalgia, because these two types of pain can be treated differently. This is where you can help, by keeping a record of your pain symptoms: where it hurts, when it is worse, how it feels, if you notice any nodules, and so on. If you believe you have both myofascial pain syndrome and fibromyalgia, it can be difficult for your doctor to properly diagnose them because they have many similar symptoms. By keeping notes and presenting them to your doctor, you can work together to come up with a diagnosis and treatment plan. (See Chapter 3, where we talk about taking notes for your diagnosis.)

Treatment of myofascial syndrome is similar in many ways to that for fibromyalgia, and we discuss them in Part 2 of this book. However, myofascial pain differs from that of fibromyalgia because it is more localized versus the diffuse pain of fibromyalgia, and treatment of myofascial pain is

CAUSES OF MYOFASCIAL PAIN SYNDROME

Although no one has come up with a definitive cause of myofascial pain syndrome, there are several theories:

• **Trauma to the muscles and skeleton**. Overuse of the muscles can cause damage to certain areas in the body and result in the development of a trigger point. Persistent trauma in the form of poor posture, having different-sized feet or leg length (which occurs in about 50 percent of people) can also contribute to the development of myofascial pain.

• **Chronic fibromyalgia pain**. Myofascial pain syndrome can arise as a result of having fibromyalgia. Here's how it happens: pain from fibromyalgia causes individuals to compensate by reducing their movements or by having an unhealthy posture, which can lead to the formation of myofascial trigger points. Severe pain caused by fibromyalgia can also cause muscle contractions around tender points, which eventually can cause trigger points to form along with tender points.

• **Depression**. At least 30 percent of people with fibromyalgia suffer from depression, which causes low serotonin levels in the brain. Since serotonin is responsible for regulating mood and pain, depression can hinder the process of regulating pain, causing myofascial pain syndrome.

often successful, whereas the pain associated with fibromyalgia has a much greater chance of being chronic.

Temporomandibular Joint Pain

Another type of pain that affects more than 75 percent of people who have fibromyalgia is temporomandibular joint disorder, or TMJ. The temporomandibular joint, which is also known as the jawbone, can cause severe pain in the jaw as well as serious and persistent headaches and other symptoms, depending on the type of TMJ. In about 25 percent of people with fibromyalgia, TMJ is chronic, while in others it is more transient.

There are two types of TMJ, joint and muscular. The majority of people with fibromyalgia who get TMJ are affected by the muscular type, which can cause headaches, difficulty opening and closing the mouth, and pain on both sides of the jaw joint. This type of TMJ affects the muscles that you use to chew and move the scalp, face, neck, and shoulders. Some physicians believe muscular TMJ is a type of fibromyalgia, although individuals can get muscular TMJ without having fibromyalgia. Causes of muscular TMJ can include stress, trauma to the muscles, or problems with the neurotransmitters in the brain.

Pain Changes Your Life

Chronic pain can impact every aspect of your life, making it difficult to cope with and manage everyday activities at home and at work, and when you go out socially. The persistent joint and muscle pain, headaches, and painful tender points prevent sleep, resulting in fatigue. When you hurt all the time, you don't feel like exercising, even though physical activity is an essential part of fibromyalgia treatment. If you have children or grandchildren, you may hurt too much to play with them. Working full-time or even part-time becomes impossible for some people who have fibromyalgia, especially women who also must care for family members.

In addition to the toll that chronic pain takes on the body, it also affects emotional and mental well-being. "It's hard to feel up when I'm in pain all the time," says Brenda, a thirty-four-year-old former teacher. Fibromyalgia forced her to stop teaching, but she now tutors a few students each week at home. "I get irritated a lot, and I feel depressed much of the time," she explains. "I used to be such an up person, and I feel like this disease has changed my personality."

The different types of pain associated with fibromyalgia can be treated, and it may take a little patience to find the most effective methods for you. We explore many different approaches in Part 2 of this book.

FATIGUE AND SLEEP PROBLEMS

"I feel like someone pulled a plug and all my energy drained out of me." That's how Amelia explains the fatigue that she lives with every day. "I wake up tired, I stay tired, and even when I sleep—and I have lots of problems with sleep—it doesn't seem to do any good. I still wake up really, really tired," says Holly, who has had fibromyalgia for five of her twenty-eight years.

Up to 90 percent of people who have fibromyalgia suffer with moderate to severe fatigue. Not everyone who has fibromyalgia experiences severe fatigue, and some make adjustments to their lives to account for their chronic tiredness. However, whether the fatigue is moderate or severe, it is persistent and does not seem to get better, even when people sleep.

Fatigue and sleep problems: these two symptoms go hand in hand. People who have fibromyalgia often wake up tired, even if they know they have slept. One theory about the sleep problem is that fibromyalgia prevents individuals from reaching REM—rapid eye movement—sleep, which is the restorative stage of sleep. Some people with fibromyalgia also experience other sleep disturbances, including sleep apnea and restless legs syndrome, which disturb what little sleep they may be getting.

When you are fatigued, you don't feel like exercising, even though physical activity helps to keep your muscles in shape, which in turn decreases pain in the long run. Thus, motivation and support are important factors for fibromyalgia patients who are challenged by fatigue. Fatigue also has another impact: it heightens emotions and stress, which can result in depression, anxiety, memory problems, and difficulties with concentration.

Sleep Problems and Pain

Sleep difficulties and pain also go hand in hand. Research shows that when your sleep is frequently interrupted, the body is unable to produce growth hormone. Without growth hormone, muscles do not heal and brain chemicals called neurotransmitters (e.g., serotonin, which is associated with mood) cannot be replenished, and pain is a result. When the body does not experience enough deep sleep, the body's systems cannot recuperate from the day's stresses, creating more sensitivity to pain.

Causes of Fatigue

Experts have several theories about the causes of fatigue in fibromyalgia, and most likely there is more than one cause for any given person who has fibromyalgia. Because the majority of people with fibromyalgia experience fatigue, some say it is the result of the pain, which all patients have. However, at least 10 percent of fibromyalgia patients do not suffer with fatigue, which suggests that pain is *a* cause but not *the* cause. In any case, here are possible causes and contributors to the fatigue that affects so many who have the syndrome.

- Some studies indicate that people with fibromyalgia have alpha-EEG anomaly, a disorder in which the brain engages in sudden activity during periods of deep sleep. These periods of increased brain activity, which can be seen on monitors as alpha waves, can cause people to wake up feeling less rested.

- Restless legs syndrome is also common among people who have fibromyalgia, affecting about 20 to 40 percent of patients. In fact, a new study (October 2010) found restless legs syndrome is ten times more common in fibromyalgia patients. This is a painful condition in which people keep moving and twitching their legs to stop the pain, which can include feelings of burning, crawling, or like the skin is being pulled. This activity typically occurs at night between the hours of 10 p.m. and 4 a.m., but it can happen during the day as well. Patients can experience these feelings for an hour or longer, making it impossible to sleep. Restless legs syndrome can be worsened by long periods of inactivity, which is another reason to exercise. The syndrome typically affects the lower legs and calves, but it can also impact the feet and arms.

- Fibromyalgia patients who suffer from extreme fatigue may have chronic fatigue syndrome, a condition diagnosed if you have experienced intense fatigue for six months or longer. More than 75 percent of people who have chronic fatigue syndrome have symptoms similar to those of fibromyalgia, and so these two conditions are often confused with one another. (See "Chronic Fatigue Syndrome" in Chapter 4.)

• Mitochondrial dysfunction is a relatively new possible explanation for the severe fatigue that many fibromyalgia patients experience. The mitochondria are tiny organs (organelles) in cells that convert nutrients and oxygen into energy for the body. Many people with fibromyalgia seem to have malfunctioning mitochondria, which means they are not producing enough energy.

• Do you stop breathing for several seconds or even longer while you are sleeping? You may not be aware of it—you may need a partner to tell you it is happening—but 80 percent of people with fibromyalgia suffer from this condition, known as sleep apnea. In sleep apnea, a person stops breathing for a few seconds or even as long as a minute. These breathing gaps are often caused by a collapse in the airway associated with snoring or being overweight, but they can also be the result of a defect in the central nervous system. In this case, the signals in the brain that tell the lungs to breathe are somehow disrupted. People who have this type of sleep apnea usually remember waking up. Regardless of which type of sleep apnea a person has, it can leave him or her feeling fatigued and thus susceptible to feeling more pain.

• Periodic limb movement disorder (PLMD) often occurs along with restless legs syndrome. In fact, 80 percent of people who have fibromyalgia and restless legs syndrome also have PLMD. Unlike restless legs syndrome, PLMD occurs only during nighttime deep sleep and it can become very physical, even violent. People with PLMD may move their feet, knees, or thighs rhythmically at intervals of between 5 and 60 seconds. The most common movements are flexes of the big toe, flexion of the knees, or fanning of the toes. People with PLMD report insomnia and fatigue.

IRRITABLE BOWEL SYNDROME

Up to 70 percent of fibromyalgia patients also have irritable bowel syndrome (IBS), a condition that affects the large intestine (bowel). It is called "irritable" because the bowel is extremely sensitive to muscle contractions that cause symptoms such as diarrhea, constipation, gas, and abdominal pain. One thing that makes IBS like fibromyalgia is that it, too, is a functional disorder, because there is no clear structural or chemical cause for the condition.

If you have both of these conditions, it is important for you to understand how they impact each other so you and your healthcare provider can find effective ways to deal with them, hopefully with options that treat symptoms of both conditions. Research shows that people who have both fibromyalgia and IBS experience symptoms that are 38 percent more severe than those who have only one of these illnesses. The challenge is that IBS tends to worsen fibromyalgia pain and fatigue, while fibromyalgia tends to increase the severity and frequency of IBS symptoms.

Like fibromyalgia, the cause of IBS is not known. What scientists do know is that IBS tends to occur after a stressful or traumatic event, such as getting a divorce, a death in the family, or starting a new job. Specific foods, such as chocolate or milk products, are suspected of triggering the disease, as are certain odors or medications. Some research also indicates that IBS may be caused by a problem with neurotransmitters in the brain, similar to what may occur in fibromyalgia.

Because both fibromyalgia and IBS involve extreme sensitivity to pain—pain in the gastrointestinal tract in IBS and in muscles and skin in fibromyalgia—scientists suggest that both conditions are caused by problems with the brain's ability to process pain messages.

IBS is a life-disrupting condition. You need to have ready access to a bathroom, because you never know when nature will call—and urgently. Some people who have IBS have needed to stop working or participating in social activities. The symptoms of diarrhea and constipation can fluctuate, coming and going without apparent reason and can be severe at times. People with IBS seem to have an overactive bowel that contracts continuously, which can cause extreme urgency or fecal incontinence, as well as cramping and bloating. Other symptoms may include lack of appetite and nausea.

You can help your doctor make a diagnosis and determine a treatment strategy if you keep a record of the foods and beverages that you consume and any reactions you have to them. Treatments are discussed in Part 2 of this book.

MULTIPLE CHEMICAL SENSITIVITY

Does the smell of perfume make you feel queasy? Do you feel dizzy whenever you walk into a furniture or fabric store? You may have multiple chemical sensitivity (MCS), a syndrome that causes people to be hypersensitive to certain smells and chemicals, as well as to certain environmental triggers, such as loud sounds, temperature, and light.

Generally, MCS affects between 17 and 34 percent of Americans on a yearly basis, but people who have fibromyalgia tend to be at increased risk. Research indicates that up to two-thirds of people who suffer from fibromyalgia also have MCS.

MCS can be insidious: first you discover you are sensitive

to one certain smell, then as time passes you find that while your sensitivity to the first trigger increases, you also develop sensitivities to other odors or stimuli. People with MCS are typically sensitive to perfumes, pesticides, fuels, carpeting, building materials, and food additives, as well as many other chemicals. MCS syndrome can cause symptoms throughout your body, including your respiratory system, skin, gastrointestinal tract, immune system, and neurological system.

Symptoms of MCS can range in severity from mild to severe and can come and go. These symptoms are associated with the condition:

Nausea and diarrhea
Itchy eyes and throat
Abdominal cramps
Aching muscles and joints
Earache
Fatigue and difficulty sleeping
Scalp pain
Difficulty breathing
Headaches and migraines
Difficulty concentrating

Although the cause of MCS is not known, many researchers believe it is purely a psychological condition, while others think it is very similar to fibromyalgia. A few theories regarding its cause include abnormal electrical activity in the brain that makes people overly sensitive, and that MCS is the result of anxiety, panic, and depression.

FIBROFOG

Are you having trouble remembering where you put your keys or what you had for breakfast this morning? Are you having difficulty concentrating, focusing on a conversation, or following simple directions? You may have fibrofog, a term used to describe the various cognitive challenges that many fibromyalgia patients experience during their illness. (A new term has been introduced to describe this mental condition: dyscognition.) These periods of "fogginess" tend to be more severe during flare-ups of pain, but they can occur at any time and vary in severity.

When fibrofog rolls in, it can last for a few days, although in severe cases it can last for weeks or even months. Fibrofog is one of the most common yet unrecognized symptoms of fibromyalgia. While it appears that people who suffer with fibrofog have no real problems with mental capacities, something causes their brain to have difficulty completing memory tasks. One possible cause of fibrofog is sleep deprivation, which is common in fibromyalgia and which causes the brain to produce an insufficient amount of serotonin, a brain chemical that helps with memory. Another possible cause is decreased blood flow to areas of the brain that are responsible for creating short-term memories.

The presence of chronic pain can inhibit the brain's ability to create memories. An excessive amount of pain can reduce the amount of time the brain spends trying to form new memories, and it can also produce a lot of stress, which can cause short-term memory loss. Depression and memory loss are linked, as depression reduces the amount of serotonin in the brain. Low serotonin levels are also associated with learning difficulties. Some other symptoms of fibrofog are difficulty remembering simple numbers, transposing letters and numbers, trouble concentrating, difficulty retaining new information, difficulty remembering plans, and trouble with language.

Besides being frustrating, having fibrofog also is associated with increased fatigue, more difficulty sleeping, and greater amount of pain. People with fibrofog can get confused about what medications they should be taking and forget where they are while out driving. Therefore it is important to report symptoms of fibrofog to your healthcare provider and to find ways to keep things in your life simple to help alleviate extra confusion. We talk about some tips in Chapter 11.

DEPRESSION

Experts estimate that at least 30 percent of fibromyalgia patients also have clinical depression and that 50 percent of those with fibromyalgia will experience severe depression at some time during their lives. When you are depressed, so many things in your life can seem worse: your pain, sleep problems, mental confusion, and fatigue, just to name a few. People with fibromyalgia may experience depression because they feel alone and misunderstood, especially if people close to them do not understand and support them during their trying times.

Depression is believed to be caused by low levels of serotonin and other chemicals in the brain. These neurotransmitters are responsible for sending signals to different parts of the brain, regulating mood, manipulating pain sensations, and other functions. When neurotransmitter levels are very low, they can cause feelings of depression. Sleep deprivation can also cause low neurotransmitter levels.

Another cause of depression in fibromyalgia may be genetic. A large number of people who have both depression and fibromyalgia also have a family history of depression.

The impact of depression on fibromyalgia can be quite profound, so it is critical that you seek treatment. Medications and alternative therapies are available to treat symptoms of depression. Depression can cause you to not exercise, to eat right, or to take your medications. You may isolate yourself, adding loneliness to depression. Although studies show that depression does not directly make fibromyalgia symptoms worse, it can cause behavioral changes that can have a negative impact on the course of the syndrome.

OTHER SYMPTOMS OF FIBROMYALGIA

Here is a brief explanation of some other symptoms of fibromyalgia. As you can see, fibromyalgia is a complex syndrome. It is important for you to tell your healthcare provider about any and all symptoms that you experience to better help you manage this condition. Again, suggested treatment options for symptoms of fibromyalgia are discussed in Part 2 of this book.

- **Chest pain.** The chest pain associated with fibromyalgia is called costochondritis, an inflammation of the cartilage that joins the ribs to the sternum, or central chest bone. Costochondritis affects about 60 to 70 percent of fibromyalgia patients, and it can manifest as intense stabbing or aching pain in your rib cage and chest that lasts for weeks or months. If this pain is making it difficult for you to breathe, sleep, or perform everyday tasks, you need to talk to your doctor. Although chest pain is usually nothing serious, occasionally it indicates other problems. The cause is unknown, but experts have several theories. One is that it is related to the tender points on the chest; another is that repetitive activity, such as leaning forward over a computer or a table places stress on the chest muscles. It may also be associated with myofascial pain syndrome. Costochondritis can be debilitating, making it difficult to sleep, sit in certain positions, or participate in certain activities.

- **Urinary problems.** Numerous urinary tract and pelvic symptoms can accompany fibromyalgia, and although they can affect both women and men, women are more likely to experience them. Urinary frequency and urgency—feeling a constant or persistent urge to urinate and having trouble holding it in—are common problems, and they hold some women captive in their homes, who are afraid to go out because they need to use the bathroom so often. These symptoms can be accompanied by pelvic pain or discomfort. Urinary incontinence, or the inability to control urination, is a frustrating problem, especially for many women. The cause of urinary incontinence with fibromyalgia is unknown, but it may be related to fatigue or weakened bladder muscles. Other related problems may include dysuria (pain while urinating) and dyspareunia (painful sexual intercourse).

• **Shortness of breath.** Research shows that feeling an urgent need for more air, or shortness of breath (also known as dyspnea) can affect up to 50 percent of fibromyalgia patients, according to a study in the *Journal of Musculoskeletal Pain.* In that study, even though the fibromyalgia patients reported feeling shortness of breath, the investigators found that they were exhaling the same amount of air as the healthy controls in the study. Thus the study's authors speculated that chest pain may be responsible for the feeling of breathlessness, even though there was no evidence to support it. Other research has shown low blood flow in the brain stem area of patients with fibromyalgia, which could be a factor. Chaotic breathing, in which people take very small, rapid breaths, may occur in about 50 percent of fibromyalgia patients. This kind of poor breathing pattern can exacerbate many other fibromyalgia symptoms, including pain, sleep problems, dizziness, headache, and others. Deep breathing exercises may be helpful.

• **Skin problems.** Between 70 and 80 percent of people with fibromyalgia suffer from skin problems, including dry itchy skin, hypersensitive skin that is sore or tender even when you touch it lightly (allodynia), rashes, and mottled skin. Dry skin can be so severe that the skin peels and causes pain and discomfort. Itchy skin can lead to excessive scratching and the development of sores or infections, while exposure of mottled skin to sunlight can cause the skin to become red and swollen. Doctors do not know why fibromyalgia patients experience so many skin problems. Overly sensitive skin and itchiness may be associated with misdirected pain signals from the brain, and mottled skin may be the result of an overactive pituitary gland in the brain. For some reason, people with fibromyalgia have an excessive amount of melanin (the substance that produces skin pigment).

• **Dysmenorrhea.** Also known as painful menstruation, this disorder can cause excruciating pain in the abdomen, pelvis, and other areas of the body during menstruation. Between 70 and 90 percent of women with fibromyalgia experience painful periods and 45 percent of these women have dysmenorrhea. Researchers believe dysmenorrhea in fibromyalgia is the result of increased sensitivity to pain. Having dysmenorrhea can make it even more difficult for women to get relief from their fibromyalgia pain.

• **Dizziness.** It is believed that the dizziness experienced by many people who have fibromyalgia is related to a condition called neurally mediated hypotension. People with fibromyalgia frequently have difficulty regulating their blood pressure. Normally, a person's heart rate increases and the blood vessels constrict when they stand up from a seated position.

In neurally mediated hypotension, a person's heart rate drops instead, preventing needed blood from being pumped around the body. This results in dizziness, fainting spells, and falls. Make sure you report dizziness symptoms to your doctor.

- **Anxiety.** About 20 percent of fibromyalgia patients experience anxiety, and it often occurs in the months following receiving a diagnosis. Anxiety is believed to be caused by chemical changes in the brain. When these chemicals (neurotransmitters, like serotonin) are out of balance, they can cause people to feel anxiety. Research suggests that fibromyalgia patients experience anxiety because they have low levels of serotonin, which is also associated with pain and depression. Feelings of anxiety can be accompanied by muscle tension, sweating, twitching, headaches, nausea, sleep disturbances, irritability, and lack of concentration. Prolonged feelings of anxiety can increase the severity of other fibromyalgia symptoms, including migraine, muscle pain, and depression.

SYMPTOMS OF FIBROMYALGIA IN CHILDREN

A common symptom that may alert you to the possibility that your child has fibromyalgia is if they experience sleep problems. If your child is having trouble falling asleep or is not getting enough sleep most days of the week, he or she is at particular risk for developing fibromyalgia syndrome. Other "red flags" include a child who catches colds easily or one who constantly feels fatigued or says he or she does not feel well.

Another symptom to watch out for is "growing pains." About 25 to 40 percent of children experience so-called growing pains—throbbing pain in the legs that typically occur late in the day or wake up children in the middle of the night. Such pains usually occur among children ages 3 to 5 years and later in 8- to 12-year-olds. These pains occur in the muscles and not the joints, and are located in the front of the thighs, in the calves, or behind the knees. For many children, these pains are likely the result of overuse from physical activity, but for some it may indicate fibromyalgia. If your child experiences persistent or excessive pain, it's time to consult your doctor. (In Chapter 10 we discuss "Raising a Child Who Has Fibromyalgia.")

CHAPTER THREE

Finding Healthcare Providers

You have probably heard stories, or perhaps you are the "subject" of such a story yourself: people who spend years going from doctor to doctor, explaining their symptoms each time, only to walk away without a diagnosis but with a dose of frustration. Then there are individuals who are suffering with what they believe are symptoms of fibromyalgia and who are trying to treat themselves because they have heard the stories about people who spend years searching for a diagnosis, and they don't want to be a part of that search. They do not want to pile more frustration onto an already life-disrupting condition.

Part of the problem can be that these individuals are not going to the "right" doctors—those who are knowledgeable about the signs and symptoms of fibromyalgia. Research indicates that many patients are not satisfied with the quality of their medical care for fibromyalgia. Patients who are not happy describe their doctors as skeptical or not sufficiently knowledgeable about their illness. Don't let this happen to you! Physicians who are knowledgeable about fibromyalgia and who are supportive of their patients **do** exist, and in this chapter we hope to help you find one or more who can assist you on your quest for a diagnosis and a treatment plan that provides a better quality of life.

If you have the signs and symptoms of fibromyalgia (see

Chapter 2), you need to work closely with a knowledgeable healthcare provider to get an accurate diagnosis and, once you have one, develop an effective treatment plan. If you have already been diagnosed with fibromyalgia, it is critical that you maintain a good working relationship with a physician whom you trust.

In this chapter we explore two critical steps you need to take before you can begin treatment for fibromyalgia: how to find the healthcare providers you need to help you diagnose and treat your signs and symptoms; and what it takes to get a diagnosis. Once you have handled these two challenges, you will be ready to move on to the treatment and relief that you need and deserve.

HOW YOU CAN HELP YOUR DOCTOR MAKE A DIAGNOSIS

While you are looking for Dr. Right, you can also be preparing for your first visit with him or her by keeping accurate records of your signs and symptoms. Possibly the best way to do this is to keep a chart of your symptoms with a separate page for each one. Make notes on each page whenever something occurs related to that symptom so you will have a detailed explanation of your condition when you meet with your doctor. Don't think to yourself, "Oh, I'll remember that I started getting bad headaches on March 8, I don't need to write it down." Please write it down. There are some other things you should take note of as well.

- Rate the level of severity of your symptoms and when the level changes; for example, changes in bowel symptoms, level of fatigue, level of pain and where.

- Record each new symptom and note the circumstances under which it started

- Write down any medications (OTC, prescription), nutritional supplements, and herbal remedies you use.

- If sleep disturbances are a problem, keep track of how much sleep you get, any sleep issues (e.g., restless legs, nightmares, sweats).

If you keep a good record of your symptoms, it can be an enormously helpful diagnostic tool for your doctor, and it will demonstrate to him or her that you are very interested in being a proactive participant in your health care and treatment.

FINDING THE RIGHT HEALTHCARE PROVIDERS

Fibromyalgia is a chronic condition, which means it's going to affect you for a long time. Therefore, it makes sense to find a physician who meets the three Cs: someone with whom you can work *closely*, someone with whom you are *comfortable*, and someone in whom you have *confidence* to not only make an accurate diagnosis, but to be there with you throughout the experience.

You may also want or need to have other healthcare providers on your team. Some people turn to a physical therapist, nutritionist, naturopath, or mental health professional for cognitive therapy. We will discuss how to find these healthcare practitioners as well. But first let's get you a "main" doctor!

Choosing Your "Main" Doctor

Your primary care physician is a good place to begin your search for a doctor to handle your diagnostic and treatment needs. He or she may be a family doctor or an internal medicine physician, someone who specializes in the study and treatment of disease in adults. Your primary care physician can make an initial assessment of your symptoms (don't forget to bring your notebook!) and refer you to a specialist.

The best possible choice for getting an accurate diagnosis and an effective treatment and management plan would be to consult a healthcare professional who is familiar with fibromyalgia. The three specialists who can best meet this goal are rheumatologists, neurologists, and pain specialists, all of whom we explain in detail below. If you have a specialist for fibromyalgia, he or she can report back to your primary care doctor if you like, or you may choose to have the specialist as your "main" doctor.

Whomever you choose to be your main doctor, he or she should always be in communication with all of your other physicians so everyone has your latest medical information, including any changes in medication. Effective communication among your main doctor, other healthcare providers, and yourself, is essential to ensure that you get the best health care possible.

Rheumatologists

Rheumatologists are medical doctors who specialize in rheumatic conditions and diseases, which include, but are

DID YOU KNOW?

A board-certified physician must complete three years of premedical education, four years of medical school that grants him or her a medical doctor or doctor of osteopathy degree, and at least three years of specialty training in an accredited residency program. Is your doctor board-certified?

not limited to, rheumatoid arthritis, osteoarthritis, osteoporosis, fibromyalgia, gout, and lupus. Rheumatology is a sub-
specialty in the area of internal medicine and focuses on the
diagnosis and treatment of illnesses that affect the joints,
bones, and muscles. It is common for a rheumatologist to be
a patient's long-term healthcare provider since rheumatic
diseases are typically chronic conditions.

Rheumatologists must complete four years of premedical
training followed by four more years at a medical school,
then three years in internal or pediatric medicine. To become qualified rheumatologists, they must complete two to
three years of specialized education and training in rheumatic disease and treatment and then pass exams to become
certified by the American Board of Internal Medicine.

A rheumatologist would likely be your best choice for
helping you with fibromyalgia, since it is a rheumatic-related
condition. Unlike other healthcare professionals, rheumatologists are very familiar with the signs and symptoms of
fibromyalgia. They are better able to rule out other rheumatic
conditions that mimic fibromyalgia and are also more used
to all the diagnostic tests they may need to help find the
cause of your fibromyalgia symptoms.

During an examination by a rheumatologist, you can expect for him or her to evaluate your bones, muscles, and
joints for areas of muscle pain as noted in the new American
College of Rheumatology (ACR) guidelines for fibromyalgia, redness and swelling, stiffness, and range of motion. To
help develop a diagnosis, rheumatologists typically rely on a
number of diagnostic test procedures, including x-rays, MRI,
electromyography, bone density tests, and aspiration of fluid
from the joints. (These procedures are discussed in detail in
Chapter 4 on "Getting a Diagnosis.")

There are a substantial number of qualified rheumatologists in the United States. If you need help finding a rheumatologist in your area, you can contact the American College
of Rheumatology (www.rheumatology.org) and their Web

site provides information on how to access individual rheumatologists around the United States and the world.

Neurologists

These specialists diagnose and treat disorders that affect both the central (brain and spinal cord) and peripheral (nerves, muscles, nerve roots) nervous systems. They can perform tests and examinations on different parts of the nervous system to diagnose and treat various conditions, including fibromyalgia, back pain, headache, muscle disorders, and reflex sympathetic dystrophy syndrome. In the United States, all neurologists are licensed by the American Board of Psychiatry and Neurology or by the American Board of Medical Specialties.

Neurologists can be an integral part of your diagnosis and treatment process, because many of the symptoms of fibromyalgia can be related to central nervous system problems, including any malfunctions in how the brain processes pain signals. An examination by a neurologist will likely include an assessment of the nerves in your head and neck, reflexes, memory and cognition, speech and language, muscle strength and movement, and balance. He or she will likely perform blood tests to rule out conditions that are often confused with fibromyalgia, like rheumatoid arthritis. You may also undergo a lumbar puncture (spinal tap) or other diagnostic test that can show how your nerves and muscles are performing, such as an MRI (magnetic resonance imaging), CT (computed tomography) scan, EEG (electroencephalography), or EMG (electromyography), all of which we mention in Chapter 4 where we discuss getting a diagnosis.

Pain Specialists

Practitioners in this area are usually board-certified anesthesiologists, neurologists, physiatrists, psychiatrists, or oncologists. Look for professionals who have received their credentials from the American Board of Anesthesiology, the American Board of Physical Medicine and Rehabilitation, the American Board of Psychiatry and Neurology, or the American Board of Pain Medicine.

Orthopedists

This specialty involves the diagnosis, treatment, and surgical repair of bone injuries, but it also covers treatment of problems associated with muscles, joints, tendons, ligaments, and cartilage.

Psychologists/Psychiatrists

These mental health specialists can diagnose and provide therapy for problems related to pain, depression, anxiety, fatigue, and mood swings. You can consult these professionals either on a one-on-one basis or in a group session.

Questions to Consider When Selecting a Doctor

Generally, there are questions you need to ask yourself and those you need to ask about the doctor. First ask yourself:

- Do you prefer to be treated by a female or male doctor? It is important to feel comfortable with the physician you choose and to feel like you can discuss your health issues and concerns without embarrassment.

- Do you prefer that your doctor be younger, older, or about the same age as you?

- Do you have a preference as to where the doctor went to school and/or interned?

- Do you have a doctor preference based on culture and/or language?

Here are some questions to consider about the doctor:

- Is the doctor board-certified?

- Where does the doctor have hospital privileges?

- Does the doctor accept your insurance?

- Is the office conveniently located and are the office hours acceptable to you?

- Is the doctor part of a group of physicians? Would you be asked to see a colleague if your doctor is not available? Is this acceptable to you?

Once you have narrowed down your choice, make an appointment for an initial consultation and physical examination. This will be the time to be prepared with questions and to see if you feel comfortable with the doctor. You may even want to bring along an understanding family member, partner, or friend for moral support. Having a second set of eyes and ears with you can give you a different perspective on the doctor.

Questions you might consider asking during your initial consultation (along with a few you will ask yourself) include:

- How does the doctor feel about alternative/complementary therapies?

- Does the doctor seem to really care about you as a person and about your concerns?

- Do you feel comfortable talking with the doctor?

• Does he or she answer your questions?

• Do the office hours fit your schedule and lifestyle?

• Which hospital is the doctor associated with?

• Which outside labs or other facilities might you have
  to go to for tests?

Whew! Once you have considered the answers to all
your questions and thought about your experience with the
doctor, we hope you have found one who makes you feel
comfortable while you work together to improve your life
with fibromyalgia.

CHOOSING ALTERNATIVE HEALTH PRACTITIONERS

At some point, you may want to consult and get treatment
from alternative health practitioners, such as acupuncturists,
massage therapists, biofeedback therapists, naturopaths,
chiropractors, herbalists, and others. (We discuss physical
therapists in Chapter 6 on Exercise and Movement Therapies.) Some of these specialists must be licensed in certain
states and not in others, and some practices are regulated
while others are not.

One way to select an alternative health practitioner is to
ask the doctor you are seeing about your fibromyalgia for a
referral or suggestion; another is to contact a national organization that governs or handles that specialty. You can also
check to see if there is a school in your area that teaches or
trains practitioners in the area you need. For example, massage schools, acupuncture schools, and naturopathic colleges
would be a good place to start for referrals or information
about these three areas of natural medicine practitioners. In
some cases, such as massage schools, they may offer dis-

counted rates if you work with a student practitioner (under the guidance of a "master," of course!).

While some of the questions you would ask when choosing a physician may not apply when seeking an alternative health provider, some of them do. You will want to know whether the individual has worked with fibromyalgia patients before, where he or she received training, which certifications, licenses, or other professional affiliations they should have, and if possible, if you can talk with other people they have treated. For additional help in finding alternative health practitioners in your area, see "Resources" for a list of national organizations, which typically provide a list of practitioners around the country, by state.

THE BOTTOM LINE

Finding healthcare providers who are knowledgeable, who make you feel comfortable, and who will work with you to diagnose and treat your fibromyalgia symptoms is an essential first step to improving your quality of life. Whether you work with one provider or you have a team of professionals you can turn to for different aspects of your treatment, we hope the relationship is a rewarding one.

CHAPTER FOUR

Getting a Diagnosis

Let's assume you have found a healthcare provider who is knowledgeable and who meets your criteria. Now it's time to get down to business: getting a diagnosis. You may have already experienced frustration in trying to get a doctor to listen to you, or perhaps you are just beginning your search. In either case, the fact is that fibromyalgia is often misunderstood by the medical community. Even though there are frequently new findings about the syndrome being added to a body of existing research, doctors still often misdiagnose this common pain disorder. As a result, some people are being given a diagnosis for chronic fatigue syndrome, arthritis, or another condition characterized by chronic pain.

The good news is that fibromyalgia is being recognized more and more by the medical community, and that there are (finally!) a new set of guidelines that healthcare providers can use, along with the criteria established back in 1990, to assist them in making a diagnosis.

So, how is a diagnosis made? Let's find out!

YOUR ROLE IN THE DIAGNOSTIC PROCESS

You can greatly help the process by being prepared for your first visit and examination if you bring the following with you:

- All of your medications, vitamins, and
  plements. Bring the bottles or other co
  are in—your doctor should see exactly
  taking.

- A list of your symptoms and information on each
  of them, such as when they occur, how often, how
  severe, when they get better or worse.

- Your family health history.

- A list of the causes of stress in your life.

- A list of questions you have about fibromyalgia and
  your overall health.

- A list of medications and supplements you took in
  the past and any reactions you had to them.

Because there is no test or procedure that can identify fibromyalgia, your symptoms are the biggest clues to begin the
search for a diagnosis. Therefore, all of the information you
can provide will greatly help your healthcare provider as he
or she takes your medical history and begins the process of
diagnosing your condition.

To help you evaluate several of the major symptoms of fibromyalgia, you might ask yourself the following questions.

How to Assess Your Fatigue Level

When you think about your loss of energy, does it:

- prevent you from participating in normal, everyday
  activities?

- make it difficult for you to make plans to do things

with your family and friends because your level of fatigue is so unpredictable?

- jeopardize your relationships with family members, friends, and others?

- make it difficult for you to get through the day?

- prevent you from exercising?

- make you still feel exhausted even if you get eight hours of sleep?

- interfere with working outside your home?

How to Assess Your Sleep Problems

When you think about your sleep patterns, do you:

- wake up many times during the night?

- typically wake up in the middle of the night?

- find it very difficult to fall asleep?

- stay awake for 10 minutes or longer whenever you wake up during the night?

- get much less sleep than you used to (before developing fibromyalgia)?

- experience restless legs syndrome

How to Assess Your Stress Level

Stress can have a tremendous impact on your physical, emotional, and spiritual health. When you think about the stress in your life, does it:

- make you feel overwhelmed every day?

- leave you feeling anxious when you wake up in the morning?

- make it difficult for you to concentrate on everyday tasks at home and/or at work?

- cause you to feel angry or irritable?

- affect your appetite (either eating more or less)?

- make it difficult for you to sleep?

- make you feel little or no interest in things you used to enjoy?

How to Assess Your Level of Depression

Your doctor will likely ask about your feelings of depression. To be prepared for his or her questions, think about whether you experience:

- a loss of interest in everyday activities and/or activities you used to enjoy?

- thoughts of dying or suicide?

- disturbed sleep patterns?

- mood swings?

- trouble concentrating?

- feelings of worthlessness or excessive guilt?

- fatigue?

- depressed thoughts or irritability?

- a desire to stay home all the time?

- agitation or the opposite—a slowing down of physical activity?

DIAGNOSTIC GUIDELINES: 1990 AND 2010

As we mentioned in Chapter 1, the American College of Rheumatology established guidelines in 1990 to help physicians identify and diagnose fibromyalgia. Many healthcare providers have voiced dissatisfaction with these original criteria for fibromyalgia pain, and some doctors have ignored them completely when evaluating patients. Then in 2010, the American College of Rheumatology issued new (but still preliminary) criteria that many physicians find to be an easier tool to evaluate patients and to come up with a diagnosis, which is great news both for doctors and for people who have been looking for answers.

Although the 2010 criteria have not been given "official" status yet (lengthy reviews are needed first), doctors have the option to use either set of criteria to help with their diagnosis. Both sets of criteria are presented and explained here.

You can see that physicians have a lot of information to deal with, and that's why we cannot emphasize enough that *your input is critical in helping to get a diagnosis*. Become

THE "ORIGINAL" CRITERIA FOR FIBROMYALGIA PAIN

The 1990 American College of Rheumatology criteria for fibromyalgia are:

- History of widespread pain that has been present for at least three months. Widespread is defined as pain in both sides of the body and pain that occurs above and below the waist. Axial skeletal pain (occurring in the cervical spine, anterior chest, thoracic spine, or lower back) must also be present.

- Pain (not just tenderness) in 11 of 18 tender points when firm finger pressure is applied. The points are bilateral (appear on both sides of the body) and are located at the following sites:
  - Back of the head (where the neck muscles attach to the base of the skull)
  - Between the shoulder blades, midway between the neck and shoulders
  - Top of the shoulders (muscles over left and right upper inner shoulder blade)
  - Front sides of the neck
  - Upper chest (upper breastbone)
  - Outer elbows
  - Upper hips
  - Sides of the hips
  - Inner knees

PRELIMINARY CRITERIA FOR FIBROMYALGIA 2010

Patients meet the diagnostic criteria for fibromyalgia if they meet the following three conditions:

- A score of 7 or higher on the widespread pain index (WPI) and 5 or higher on the Symptom Severity (SS) Scale; or 3 to 6 on the WPI and 9 or higher on the SS

- They have experienced symptoms at a similar level of severity for at least 3 months

- Patients do not have a condition that can otherwise explain the pain

Details of the WPI Score

Clinicians determine the areas in which the patient has had pain over the last week. A total of 19 areas are considered, so the score will be between 0 and 19:

Shoulder girdle, left and/or right
Upper arm, left and/or right
Lower arm, left and/or right
Hip (buttock), left and/or right
Upper leg, left and/or right
Lower leg, left and/or right
Jaw, left and/or right
Chest
Abdomen
Upper back
Lower back
Neck

Details of the SS Score

Score three symptoms—fatigue, waking unrefreshed, cognitive symptoms—on a scale ranging from 0 to 3, using the following:

0 = no problem
1 = slight or mild problems generally mild
   or intermittent
2 = moderate, considerable problems, often present
   and/or at a moderate level
3 = severe; pervasive, continuous, life-disturbing
   problems

Additional Somatic Symptoms

Patients rate how many other symptoms they may experience *in addition to* the three mentioned above. The score for these additional symptoms is then added to the SS score from the three major symptoms. Thus, the final SS score can be between 0 and 12. Patients rate additional symptoms as follows:

0 = no symptoms
1 = few symptoms
2 = a moderate number of symptoms
3 = great number of symptoms

Those additional symptoms may include muscle pain, irritable bowel syndrome, muscle weakness, headache, pain/cramps in the abdomen, numbness/tingling, dizziness, insomnia, depression, constipation, pain in the upper abdomen, nausea, nervousness, chest pain, blurry vision, fever, diarrhea, dry mouth, itching, wheezing, Raynaud's phenomenon, hives, ringing in ears, vomiting, heartburn, oral ulcers, loss of/change in taste, seizures, dry eyes, shortness of breath, loss of appetite, rash, sensitivity to the sun, hearing difficulties, easy bruising, hair loss, frequent urination, painful urination, bladder spasms.

familiar with both sets of criteria so you and your doctor can better work together on getting help for you.

Your healthcare provider will perform a physical examination that may include use of the criteria from either of the guidelines we have listed here. His or her findings will be combined along with your reported symptoms to form a more complete picture of your condition. Then there is the task of "ruling out" other similar or related conditions.

"RULING OUT" TO GET A DIAGNOSIS

Along with a thorough evaluation of your symptoms, your healthcare provider will need to conduct various tests and studies as part of the diagnostic process. These may include blood tests, imaging tests, and electrophysiological studies of the muscles and nerves to rule out illnesses that have similar symptoms, such as rheumatoid arthritis, chronic fatigue syndrome, lupus, Lyme disease, hypothyroidism, and muscle diseases (e.g., myofascial pain syndrome, discussed in Chapter 2). This is the major reason why it is difficult to diagnose fibromyalgia, why it can take years to arrive at a diagnosis (unless you can find a knowledgeable healthcare provider early in your search), and why so many people who are suffering with symptoms end up also having to deal with numerous doctors, tests, and procedures.

Let's take a closer look at some of the more common

conditions that your healthcare provider may need to "rule out" during the diagnostic process and some of the clues he or she will be looking for during the process. You will see that there are no definitive signs or symptoms for any of these conditions, which can make the search all that more difficult. It is also true that a person can have both fibromyalgia and another condition at the same time. However, you can greatly help your physician make a diagnosis if you carefully and accurately keep track of your symptoms and any changes as they occur, because all of these things are clues to uncovering a diagnosis.

Is It Chronic Fatigue Syndrome?

Research indicates that up to 70 percent of patients who have fibromyalgia also fit the criteria for chronic fatigue syndrome (CFS). People who have chronic fatigue syndrome, however, generally do not meet the criteria for fibromyalgia. Pain is the notable characteristic of fibromyalgia, while fatigue is the hallmark of CFS. Clinicians can look for a factor called substance P, which may be found in high levels in the spinal fluid of fibromyalgia patients while CFS patients may not. People who have CFS are more likely to experience fever, sore throat, and swollen glands than people who have fibromyalgia. Another distinguishing factor is that aerobic exercise often improves muscle function and reduces pain in fibromyalgia patients, but in people who have CFS, exercise can be impossible to do and generally makes symptoms worse.

Is It Lupus?

Lupus, also called systemic lupus erythematosus (SLE) is a chronic autoimmune disease that affects the joints, kidneys, skin, heart, and other tissues and organs throughout the body. It is most commonly seen in women of childbearing age, but it can occur in women of any age, as well as in men. African-American women are about three times more likely to have the disease than Caucasian women, and it is also more common in Hispanic, Asian, and Native American women.

The symptoms vary in severity from mild to severe and from patient to patient over time. However, the most common symptoms of the disease are painful swollen joints, fatigue, rash (often a "butterfly" rash across the cheeks and under the eyes), fever, a general feeling of not being well, and muscle pain. Other symptoms may include hair loss, chest pain that gets worse when breathing deeply, sensitivity to sunlight, sores in the mouth or nose, swollen glands, and weight loss.

Is It Lyme Disease?

Lyme disease is a progressive, systemic condition that is caused by the bacteria *Borrelia burgdorferi,* which is typically transmitted to people when they are bitten by an infected deer tick. About 23,000 people get Lyme disease each year. At first, symptoms are similar to those you would expect with the flu, such as fever, headache, fatigue, muscle pain, and malaise. These symptoms usually go away without treatment. Perhaps you've heard that everyone who has Lyme disease gets a characteristic "bull's-eye" rash, but do not count on this sign to know you have the disease. Experts vary greatly as to what percentage of people who have Lyme disease actually develop this rash (the range is 10 percent to 80 percent).

If Lyme disease is not treated, it may progress to cause arthritis and impact the central nervous system and heart. This occurs in about 10 percent of people with the infection. This stage may also be resolved without treatment. If the disease progresses to the third stage, which can take months to years after getting bitten, it affects the musculoskeletal, cardiovascular, ophthalmologic, and central nervous systems. If this occurs, symptoms can include inflammation of the joints causing pain, inflammation of the cornea causing decreased vision, inflammation of the heart muscle (myocarditis), multiple rashes, brain dysfunction resulting in memory loss, and other complications.

Is It Rheumatoid Arthritis?

Rheumatoid arthritis is a chronic autoimmune disease in which the lining of the joint capsule (synovium) and the tendons become inflamed. In autoimmune diseases such as rheumatoid arthritis, the immune system attacks healthy cells, causing damage and inflammation. Signs and symptoms of rheumatoid arthritis are chronic pain, permanent joint damage, and loss of joint function. But rheumatoid arthritis does not just affect the joints. Because it is a multisystemic disease, it can also attack any number of organs, including the skin, heart, lungs, and eyes. An estimated 2.1 million people in the United States have rheumatoid arthritis, and about 70 percent of them are women.

One clue your doctor may look for is the rheumatoid factor, an antibody that is found in high levels in about 70 to 80 percent of patients who have rheumatoid arthritis. However, not everyone who has high levels of rheumatoid factor has rheumatoid arthritis, and not all patients who have rheumatoid arthritis have elevated levels of the factor.

Here are some other clues. In most cases, people with rheumatoid arthritis have joint pain and stiffness that is more severe after they have been inactive, such as when they get up in the morning. The joints that are most often affected are the hands, wrists, cervical spine (neck), shoulders, elbows, hips, and knees. Another clue: joint pain and stiffness usually develop first in the small joints in the fingers, hands, wrists, and feet. If the right wrist is affected, most likely the left one is, too. That's because joint involvement is usually symmetrical, occurring on both sides of the body.

As rheumatoid arthritis progresses, it causes damage to the

cartilage, tendons, ligaments, and bones, which can result in deformity and loss of joint function. Other symptoms of rheumatoid arthritis may also sound familiar—they are also found in fibromyalgia patients: depression, fatigue, muscle pain, weakness, and loss of appetite.

Is It Hypothyroidism?

Hypothyroidism is a condition in which the thyroid gland does not make enough thyroid hormones. Approximately 10 million people in American have this condition, and it is believed that 10 percent of women have some degree of thyroid hormone deficiency. Because the thyroid is responsible for regulating metabolism, the lack of sufficient hormones results in symptoms one would associate with a slow metabolism: fatigue, weakness, weight gain, depression, memory loss, decreased libido, dry hair, pale skin, hair loss, cold intolerance, muscle cramps, muscle aches, constipation, and abnormal menstrual cycles. Once again, many of these symptoms are right out of the list of symptoms for fibromyalgia.

Each person with hypothyroidism can have any number of these symptoms, and they can vary in intensity depending

DID YOU KNOW?

Frances Winfield Bremer, the wife of Ambassador L. Paul Bremer III, was diagnosed with fibromyalgia nearly 30 years ago. In 2007, the National Fibromyalgia Association named her its official spokesperson. She and her husband make joint media appearances to promote awareness of the syndrome and motivate more people into discovering a cure.

on how deficient the individual is and how long the body has been deprived of an adequate amount of the hormones.

TESTING FOR FIBROMYALGIA

The laboratory tests and any procedures that your doctor performs will add more clues to the overall picture. Although the exact diagnostic approach a doctor takes differs for each patient depending on an individual's symptoms and results of the physical exam, the following tests and procedures are among the ones you may encounter.

- **Complete blood count (CBC).** This test measures the levels of red cells, white cells, hemoglobin, and platelets, among other values that involve these factors. A CBC may show an abnormally high white blood cell count, which is an indication of an infection. A decline in red blood cell count may indicate anemia. In any case, it is good to have a baseline CBC test so any subsequent tests can be compared against it.

- **Blood calcium levels.** This test is done to determine if the level of calcium in your blood is abnormally high, which would mean you have hypercalcemia. This condition is characterized by nonspecific symptoms such as nausea, loss of appetite, muscle weakness, confusion, fatigue, and restlessness.

- **Thyroid panel.** This test is done to rule out hypothyroidism. The two most important thyroid hormones are thyroxine (T4) and triiodothyronine (T3); a third hormone is thyroid-stimulating hormone (TSH). A thyroid panel measures the levels of all three. A high TSH and normal T4 and T3 indicate mild hypothyroidism, while high TSH, low T4, and

low or normal T3 is a stronger indication of hypothyroidism.

- **Antinuclear antibody (ANA).** ANA is an abnormal
  antibody that is commonly found in the bloodstream
  of people who have lupus.

- **Rheumatoid factor.** This blood test determines
  whether there is an abnormal level of rheumatoid factor in the blood. Results of this test are not definitive,
  however, because it can be positive in healthy people
  and negative in people who have rheumatoid arthritis.

- **Erythrocyte sedimentation rate (ESR).** This test
  provides a rough index of the level of inflammation in
  the body. In people who have fibromyalgia, the ESR
  rate is usually normal, while it typically is abnormal in
  people who have rheumatoid arthritis, polymyalgia
  rheumatica, and other similar conditions.

- **X-rays.** An x-ray cannot reveal pain, but it can reveal
  some abnormalities to indicate what type of arthritis
  you may have. X-rays cannot, however, diagnose fibromyalgia.

- **Joint aspiration.** If you have fluid in a joint, your
  doctor may aspirate it—use a sterile needle and sy-
  ringe to withdraw it from the joint. An analysis of
  joint fluid can help determine the cause of joint swelling or arthritis, such as infection, rheumatoid disease,
  or gout.

- **Lumbar puncture.** Also known as a spinal tap, it
  involves inserting a needle between two vertebrae in
  your lower back to remove a sample of cerebrospinal
  fluid, which surrounds the brain and spinal cord to

protect them from injury. In people who have fibro-myalgia, an agent called substance P is often present, while it is less likely to be found in people who have chronic fatigue syndrome. A lumbar puncture causes moderate to severe headaches in about one-third of people who undergo the procedure, and the head pain can last several hours to a week or longer.

Blood Pressure and Hair Analysis Testing

Two other tests that are less common but attracting attention are the blood pressure test and hair analysis test. In the December 2006 issue of the *Journal of Clinical Rheumatology,* scientists reported on a simple test for fibromyalgia. They found that most of the fibromyalgia patients experienced pain when they had their blood pressure taken.

In the study, the researchers evaluated 20 fibromyalgia patients, 20 patients with rheumatoid arthritis, 20 who had osteoarthritis, and 20 healthy volunteers. Each study participant was asked the same questions: "When I take your blood pressure, tell me if the cuff's pressure brings forth pain." Sixty-nine percent of the fibromyalgia patients said yes, compared with only 10 percent of osteoarthritis patients, five percent of rheumatoid arthritis patients, and 2 percent of the healthy volunteers. Also, the average blood pressure value at which the fibromyalgia patients experience pain was lower than the other three groups.

Hair analysis involves examining the protein in a small sample of hair. Because hair is metabolically very active, it can reveal a variety of things about an individual, including exposure to toxins and heavy metals, and any vitamin, mineral, and other nutritional deficiencies. Another benefit of a hair analysis is that it can help your doctor determine the best treatment for you, including any dietary changes to address nutritional deficiencies.

Studies have shown that the hair samples of people with

fibromyalgia frequently have a higher level of calcium and magnesium than people without the syndrome. Some experts also believe that exposure to certain toxins, such as aspartame, accumulate in the body and are revealed in the hair. The buildup of toxins can trigger the body to create pain receptors in the muscle fibers, which can then result in chronic pain.

Hair analysis is still a controversial testing procedure. Some experts question its validity and accuracy, and suggest that the lack of standardized lab procedures may be part of the problem. However, your healthcare provider may use this analysis as part of the diagnostic process.

Other Tests

As part of the "ruling out" process, your doctor may conduct several other tests, including imaging as well as muscle and brain testing. X-rays and imaging techniques of painful areas in people who have fibromyalgia will not show any abnormalities, because the pain associated with fibromyalgia is in the muscles and tendons. However, if arthritis is the cause of your pain, for example, then imaging techniques can be helpful.

Here are four tests that physicians may order when trying to reach a diagnosis:

- **Magnetic resonance imaging (MRI).** An MRI uses electromagnetic radio waves to produce two- or three-dimensional computer images of the organs, muscles, bones, and nerves. Compared with a CT scan, an MRI produces more detailed images of soft tissues and organs. It can be used to accurately detect and locate tumors. It is also used to help diagnose multiple sclerosis, which may have symptoms similar to those of fibromyalgia. An MRI scan can be used to detect patches of tissue in the brain that confirm this disease.

- **Computed tomography (CT) scan.** This imaging technique is used to create cross-sectional images of structures in the body. Unlike an MRI, it uses x-rays that are taken at various angles and then processed through a computer to produce the images. A CT is used to detect abnormalities such as blood clots, cysts, fractures, infections, and tumors in bones, muscles, organs, and soft tissues.

- **Electroencephalogram (EEG).** This test measures the electrical activity of the brain. Because normal brain waves have recognizable patterns, any abnormalities may suggest a seizure disorder, tumors in the brain, migraines, hallucinations, or head injury. It can also indicate sleep disorders, which is a key reason why a doctor who suspects you have a sleep disorder may order an EEG.

- **Electromyography (EMG).** Also known as a nerve conduction test, it is used to assess the health and function of the muscles and nerves that control the muscles. It can be used to identify whether muscle weakness and loss of muscle strength are caused by a neurological disorder or a muscle injury. Some of the disorders it may detect include muscular dystrophy, myasthenia gravis, neuropathy, and sciatic nerve dysfunction.

AND THE DIAGNOSIS IS . . .

It may sound strange, but for many people who finally get a diagnosis of fibromyalgia after months, even years of going to doctors, and living with pain, fatigue, and uncertainty, they feel relieved, even happy. "Someone finally validated what I was going through," said Becky, a forty-one-year-old former college administrator. "It has a name. I finally feel like I can move forward. I feel hopeful." For Becky, it meant she felt confident enough to try different therapies. For others, getting a diagnosis means family and friends "finally believe me," said Pauline, who at fifty-two had been suffering for nearly five years.

We hope your journey through the diagnostic process will bring you to a resolution. Getting a diagnosis is a big beginning, because now a new journey begins—the road to healing and living well with fibromyalgia.

PART II

Take Charge of Your Life With Fibromyalgia

CHAPTER FIVE

Treating Fibromyalgia With Medication

Fibromyalgia is a complex syndrome, and so the best way to treat it is to engage a variety of treatment modalities. One of those modalities is the use of over-the-counter (OTC) and/or prescription medications, and fortunately there is quite an arsenal from which to choose. Medications can be used along with exercise—an absolutely critical part of treatment—as well as nutritional, herbal, and other alternative/ complementary methods to relieve your symptoms, help you function better, and improve your quality of life. There is so much you can do, so don't despair!

The goal of treatment with medication is to provide patients with options that work with their brain chemistry to reduce pain and fatigue, ease depression and anxiety, and improve sleep, as well as address other symptoms, so their quality of life is the very best it can be. Generally, the focus of treatment is different for each person, depending on the severity of symptoms and which symptoms are the most troublesome, although pain management is always part of the treatment regimen.

This chapter identifies both OTC and prescription medications most often used to treat symptoms of fibromyalgia, their side effects, precautions you should take when using them, and the typical dosages. We explore the three FDA-approved drugs for fibromyalgia, which include Lyrica (pregabalin), Savella (milnacipran), and Cymbalta (duloxetine), and drugs in the categories that physicians typically prescribe for fibromyalgia: analgesics, antidepressants, muscle relaxants, and antiseizure drugs.

We also take a look at a controversial approach called the Guaifenesin Protocol, which was developed by Dr. R. Paul St. Amand. Guaifenesin is an OTC drug used to clear mucus from the chest, but advocates say it has proven effective in relieving symptoms of fibromyalgia.

WHAT FIBROMYALGIA PATIENTS ARE TAKING

In May 2009, the *Journal of Women's Health* published an article that revealed how women with fibromyalgia were treating their symptoms. Researchers surveyed 434 women who had fibromyalgia and found that 93 percent were taking at least one conventional medication, with an average of 4.6 medications per person. Half of the women said they were taking antidepressant drugs, and the most commonly used were selective serotonin reuptake inhibitors (SSRIs). Only a few were taking the newly approved pregabalin.

A startling finding was that nearly 30 percent were taking nonsteroidal anti-inflammatory drugs (NSAIDs), which have not been found to be effective for treating fibromyalgia. The women also reported taking anticonvulsants, muscle relaxants, narcotics, other painkillers, benzodiazepines, and guaifenesen. Overall, the women rated the guaifenesen and opioid narcotics as being the most effective. (The women also reported taking natural supplements, which are discussed in Chapter 8.)

The researchers concluded the fact that women were taking a wide variety of medications, along with the fact that so many were taking NSAIDs that lacked evidence for effectiveness, indicates that there are few medications that provide consistent and/or reliable symptom relief.

However, the fact that there are so many treatment choices may also work to a patient's benefit, because when one medication does not provide sufficient relief, another may. And with that introduction, let's look at the medication options.

WHERE TO BEGIN

If you are like most patients with fibromyalgia, you have a laundry list of symptoms. In that case, you may want to "take it from the top," which is what many doctors suggest: focus on relieving the top one or two symptoms that are most disruptive in the patient's life. This is an important approach for several reasons. One is that it is too easy to become caught up in taking too many medications at the same time. If you try treating one symptom with more than one drug, and then another symptom with one or more drugs, you may end up taking three or more medications, and exposing yourself to possible drug interactions and side effects from each of the substances. You may then find yourself needing to take something to treat the side effects—and you have enough to worry about just relieving your main symptoms!

Another reason why treating one symptom at a time with a minimal number of medications is important is that you and your doctor can better identify which drug is working— or not working. Once you find an effective medication, it will also give you more confidence and strength to perhaps try complementary therapies, which can greatly reduce your need for medication and any associated side effects.

Every person who has fibromyalgia experiences different symptoms at varying degrees of severity and at different times. So although there is no one approach or magic bullet that will fix everything, there are plenty of options you and your healthcare provider can try! The first medication your doctor chooses may not be effective, but if you work closely with your physician and accurately report any side effects and how you feel when taking a medication, you can increase your chances of finding something that works for you. This includes telling your doctor about any other treatment approaches you are using, such as natural supplements, movement therapies, acupuncture, and other alternative approaches.

ANALGESICS

Analgesics are drugs that have been designed to relieve pain. Because pain is the most distressing and pervasive symptom of fibromyalgia, finding effective ways to relieve it is paramount. Certainly analgesics are one way to address pain, but as you'll see later in this chapter, some other types of medications can also help relieve pain.

Analgesics fall into four categories: acetaminophen, nonsteroidal anti-inflammatory drugs (NSAIDs), COX-2 inhibitors, and narcotics. Here is a review of what is available for fibromyalgia patients and how they may help. Discuss the most appropriate dosage for your needs with your healthcare provider, as it will depend on the severity of your symptoms, other medications and/or supplements you may be taking, and other symptoms you are experiencing.

Acetaminophen

Acetaminophen (e.g., Acephen, Tylenol) is the most widely used painkiller and fever fighter in the United States and the world. It is available both alone and in many combination medications. In fact, acetaminophen is often used along with narcotics for fibromyalgia patients to enhance the pain-reducing benefit. Acetaminophen relieves pain by raising the pain threshold, which means a greater amount of pain must develop before a person feels it. The FDA approved this drug in 1951. It is available both OTC and by prescription at higher doses than found on your drugstore shelves.

When used occasionally, acetaminophen rarely causes side effects. However, chronic, long-term use, which may be how some people with fibromyalgia use it, can result in liver damage. Therefore it is important to find other ways to both complement and replace the use of acetaminophen with safer options, as we discuss in Chapters 7 and 8. It is also important that you do not drink alcohol if you are taking acetaminophen. The maximum daily dose is 4,000 mg.

Nonsteroidal Anti-inflammatory Drugs (NSAIDs)

This large class of drugs, some of which are available OTC, treats both pain and inflammation. However, because fibromyalgia is not an inflammatory condition, the effectiveness of NSAIDs for treatment of this syndrome can be minimal. (They are, however, among the most commonly used drugs for fibromyalgia, as we noted above.) The more common NSAIDs and an example brand name are listed below. Long-term use of these drugs can cause bleeding in the gastrointestinal (GI) tract and ulcers. In fact, regular use of NSAIDs is the second major cause of ulcers. Use of NSAIDs also raises blood pressure, and these drugs can counteract the benefits of some blood pressure drugs.

COMMON NSAIDs

Aspirin (Bayer)
Diclofenac (Voltaren)
Diflunisal (Dolobid)
Etodolac (Lodine)
Ibuprofen (Motrin)
Indomethacin (Indocin)
Ketoprofen (Actron)
Ketorolac (Toradol)

Nabumetone (Relafen)
Naproxen (Aleve)
Oxaprozin (Daypro)
Piroxicam (Feldene)
Sulindac (Clinoril)
Tolmetin (Tolectin)

COX-2 Inhibitors

COX-2 inhibitors are a type of NSAID that selectively blocks
a specific enzyme (COX-2) that can cause stomach irritation
and GI bleeding. Therefore, Celebrex [celecoxib] is associated with less risk of GI problems than are other NSAIDs,
but that does not mean the risk is gone. At one point there
were three COX-2 inhibitors on the market (Celebrex [cele-
coxib], Bextra [valdecoxib], and Vioxx [rofecoxib]), but only
celecoxib remains, after the other two were withdrawn by
the FDA because they were linked with an increased risk of
heart attack.

Narcotics (Opioids)

Questions about the effectiveness and the appropriateness
of narcotics to treat fibromyalgia pain are ongoing. You will
see many articles that say narcotics are not effective in relieving fibromyalgia pain, while others tell stories of patients
who say they work well for them. Because of the chronic
nature of fibromyalgia, many doctors are reluctant to prescribe narcotics because of worries about dependence and/or
abuse. Other doctors are willing to work with their patients in
prescribing narcotics in a controlled fashion.

When the body senses pain, pain signals are sent by nerve
cells to certain receptors in the body. Opioids attach to opioid receptors in the brain, gastrointestinal tract, and spinal
cord, which receive some of the pain messages. The opioids

block the receptors from accepting the pain signals, which then reduces the sensation of pain.

People with moderate to severe fibromyalgia pain who have used opioids have reported relief from pain symptoms, an increased ability to function, and a reduction in the number of pain flare-ups. However, opioids are not a long-term solution to chronic muscle pain and so are recommended only for short-term use, which your doctor can determine.

Opioids are classified by the types of receptors to which they attach and how they work. There are three main types. Full agonists continue to increase in efficacy over time and work on receptors in the brain. They will not interfere with the effects of other opioids. Examples include morphine, codeine, oxycodone, methadone, and fentanyl.

Partial agonists will eventually stop being effective, and they are not efficient at blocking pain signals at brain receptors. A common example is buprenorphine. Mixed agonists-antagonists will eventually stop working as well. They also work on only one receptor site in the brain, and they should not be used with a full agonist. Examples include pentazocine and dezocine.

Opioids often cause unwanted side effects, especially if they are used for an extended time. They include drowsiness, nausea, vomiting, loss of appetite, blurry vision, sweating, constipation, and euphoria.

Ultram (tramadol) and Ultracet (tramadol plus acetaminophen) are opioids that also have SSNR (selective serotonin norepinephrine reuptake inhibitors, a type of antidepressant discussed elsewhere in this chapter) properties, so they are almost in a class by themselves. They can be used to treat moderate to severe pain, and Ultram extended-release formula is used when pain relief is needed around the clock.

What about addiction dependence? Although this can be an issue, patients who work closely with their healthcare practitioner and who explore other pain-relieving avenues can

> ## DID YOU KNOW?
>
> The potent sleeping pill Xyrem may help relieve pain in people with fibromyalgia, according to a new study presented at the annual meeting of the American Pain Society in May 2010. When compared with placebo, more than 50 percent of people who took Xyrem reported at least a 30 percent improvement in pain. Xyrem also helped with fatigue and stiffness.

usually use these drugs without a problem. Withdrawing from opioids can cause some disturbing symptoms, even among people who are not addicted. However, if you taper off slowly and under the guidance of your physician, symptoms can be minimized. Those symptoms may include diarrhea, runny nose, yawning, drug cravings, anxiety, and insomnia.

OTHER MEDICATIONS FOR PAIN

A few unlikely medications are also used to tackle the pain of fibromyalgia. One is a drug typically used to treat Parkinson's disease, called pramipexole (Mirapex). Pramipexole is a dopamine receptor agonist, which means that it stimulates the production of a chemical transmitter called dopamine in the brain. Dopamine helps to reduce the body's response to pain. Several studies have shown that 80 percent of fibromyalgia patients reported a 30 percent improvement in pain and 40 percent reported a 50 percent reduction in pain when taking pramipexole. The most common side effects are nausea and constipation.

Pindolol (Visken) is a beta-adrenergic receptor that calms the sympathetic nervous system by blocking the neurotransmitter norepinephrine. This drug may help fibromyalgia patients because they typically have excessive amounts of norepinephrine in their system. These high levels prevent receptors in the brain from being activated without getting a big boost of activity from the sympathetic nervous system, which can result in pain and stress. A study of pindolol in fibromyalgia patients found that the drug substantially improved muscle pain, muscle stiffness, and sleep problems. People who use pindolol may experience excessive perspiration.

ANTICONVULSANTS

Anticonvulsants are drugs developed to treat seizures, but they also have the ability to relieve different types of pain. The first medication approved by the Food and Drug Administration specifically for pain related to fibromyalgia was the anticonvulsant Lyrica (pregabalin). Another anticonvulsant prescribed for fibromyalgia in off-label use is Neurontin (gabapentin).

Experts theorize that anticonvulsants help relieve fibromyalgia pain because these drugs suppress the excitability of the nervous system. Fibromyalgia is believed to be caused, at least in part, by hypersensitivity of the central nervous system, with pain signals being transmitted much more often than they should be. Use of anticonvulsants may reduce those signals.

Although pregabalin has FDA approval for treatment of fibromyalgia and gabapentin does not, gabapentin is chemically very similar to pregabalin and has been shown in studies to be effective in relieving pain in fibromyalgia as well. In the April 2007 issue of *Arthritis & Rheumatism*, researchers reported that gabapentin taken for 12 weeks at 1,200 to 2,400 mg daily significantly reduced pain when compared with a placebo. The patients also said they slept significantly better and had less fatigue. Side effects included mild to moderate dizziness and sedation, which are also experienced by people who use pregabalin.

ANTIDEPRESSANTS

Antidepressants can be helpful in relieving several symptoms characteristic of fibromyalgia, including pain, depression, and poor sleep. Your doctor may recommend one or more of several different types of antidepressants, depending on your symptoms.

Selective Serotonin and Norepinephrine Reuptake Inhibitors (SNRIs)

Selective serotonin and norepinephrine reuptake inhibitors (SNRIs) can relieve pain even if you are not experiencing depression. Two of the three FDA-approved drugs to treat fibromyalgia—Cymbalta and Savella—are in this category. Doctors also prescribe Effexor to relieve fibromyalgia pain in an off-label use.

- **Cymbalta (duloxetine).** Only the second drug approved by the FDA explicitly for treatment of fibromyalgia, Cymbalta had previously been approved to manage major depressive disorder, general anxiety disorder, and diabetic peripheral nerve pain. This drug can be beneficial because it helps to elevate levels of serotonin and norepinephrine in the brain and spinal cord, where they are involved in mood symptoms and the regulation of the perception of pain. Cymbalta is approved only for adults 18 and older. This antidepressant can increase suicidal thoughts and behaviors in young adults. You should not take Cymbalta if you have uncontrolled glaucoma or have recently taken a monoamine oxidase inhibitor (MAOI).

Before starting Cymbalta, talk to your doctor if you have kidney problems, diabetes, glaucoma, high blood pressure, seizure disorders, bleeding disorders, or liver problems. Taking Cymbalta along with NSAIDs or blood thinners may increase the risk of bleeding. The most common side effects of Cymbalta are dry mouth, nausea, sleepiness, dizziness, fainting upon standing, and constipation.

- **Savella (milnacipran).** Savella is the third drug approved by the FDA for fibromyalgia. In clinical studies, Savella was better than a placebo in reducing pain, providing overall improvement in fibromyalgia symptoms, and improved physical function. The precautions associated with Savella are similar to those listed for Cymbalta. The most common side effect is nausea. In clinical trials, side effects included headache, constipation, dizziness, insomnia, hot flush, excessive sweating, vomiting, palpitations, and dry mouth. Savella can also cause a rise in blood pressure (see "Did You Know?").

- **Effexor (venlafaxine).** Treatment of fibromyalgia symptoms is an off-label use for this SNRI. Side effects are similar to those for Savella and Cymbalta.

Selective Serotonin Reuptake Inhibitors (SSRIs)

Selective serotonin reuptake inhibitors (SSRIs) such as Paxil, Zoloft, and Prozac, can improve sleep, reduce pain, and support an improved sense of well-being. Research shows that SSRIs are not as effective as SNRIs in relieving fibromyalgia symptoms.

DID YOU KNOW?

In January 2010, the consumer advocacy group Public Citizen asked the FDA to withdraw Savella from the market because of lack of effectiveness and its side effects, the same reasons European regulators rejected the drug in 2009. Public Citizen also noted that the manufacturers' studies showed 20 percent of patients taking Savella had high blood pressure compared with 7 percent of those taking a dummy pill. In terms of effectiveness, company scientists recorded 9 percent of patients on Savella had a significant reduction in pain compared with 7 percent of those taking a placebo.

Tricyclic Antidepressants

The tricyclic antidepressants are sometimes prescribed for fibromyalgia, but they tend to have more disturbing side effects (e.g., weight gain, dizziness, fatigue) than SSRIs and SNRIs. When tricyclics are taken at low doses, they do not help mood or anxiety, which are common issues in people who have fibromyalgia, but they can help by improving deep, restorative sleep.

Your physician may recommend a combination of antidepressants to address your most disturbing symptoms. Some patients find that a combination of antidepressants significantly reduces pain while also relieving depression and anxiety and helping them sleep.

MUSCLE RELAXANTS

The term "muscle relaxants" is a little inaccurate. Not all drugs classified as muscle relaxants truly relax muscles or reduce muscle spasms, because the painful area still experiences spasms. Instead, most muscle relaxants help to cover up or mask pain, working to reduce the brain's ability to sense pain, which then allows you to relax, and as a result, relaxes your muscles, too. Muscle relaxants also block the pain signals that your nerves send to the brain.

Drugs classified as muscle relaxants that are more commonly used to treat fibromyalgia include carisoprodol (Soma), cyclobenzaprine (Flexeril), orphenadrine citrate (Norflex), and tizanidine (Zanaflex). All muscle relaxants can cause side effects, and your healthcare provider should monitor you carefully while you are taking any of these medications. The most common side effects include drowsiness, constipation, and dry mouth. Muscle relaxants can be habit-forming and should not be taken for extended periods of time unless you are under a doctor's supervision.

- **Carisoprodol.** This drug is designed to reduce stiffness, pain, and muscle injury, and it is also very effective at reducing muscle spasms in fibromyalgia patients. Carisoprodol acts on the brain by blocking nerve impulses involved with pain sensations. Few studies have been done regarding its effectiveness in fibromyalgia patients, but it is generally believed to be as effective as cyclobenzaprine.

- **Cyclobenzaprine.** In one study of 120 fibromyalgia patients, cyclobenzaprine significantly reduced pain and muscle tightness, and all the patients also said they slept better when taking the drug. Their total number of tender points also declined. In a meta-analysis that included evaluation of five placebo-controlled, double-blind studies, the researchers found that patients taking cyclobenzaprine were three times as likely to report overall improvement and moderate reductions in individual symptoms, especially sleep problems. Because use of cyclobenzaprine can cause addiction and withdrawal symptoms, talk to your doctor before taking this drug. This drug generally should not be taken for longer than three months. If you have any type of heart condition, you should not use cyclobenzaprine.

- **Orphenadrine citrate.** This drug also acts on the brain to block muscle pain. It works best when combined with physical therapy and rest. In a study of 85 patients with fibromyalgia, orphenadrine reduced pain symptoms by up to 34 percent after one year of treatment. Although orphenadrine can be used for a longer time than cyclobenzaprine, it may also cause disturbing side effects, including tremors and confusion.

- **Tizanidine.** Like cyclobenzaprine and orphenadrine, tizanidine also blocks nerve impulses. However, this drug is also especially helpful in reducing muscle spasms and can also increase muscle tone. Do not use tizanidine if you are taking oral contraceptives or if you have liver or kidney disease.

SLEEP MEDICATIONS

"If I could just get some sleep!" If you suffer from insomnia, this is a common lament. Successfully treating insomnia and the resulting fatigue is a major goal of fibromyalgia patients, and some medications can help. However, sleeping pills are meant to be used on a temporary basis, not to treat chronic insomnia. Pharmaceutical sleep aids should be considered a last resort for patients who have fibromyalgia or they should be used only infrequently. To reduce the risk of side effects and of becoming reliant on any drug to help you sleep, your doctor should prescribe medications for two weeks or less.

Sleeping pills are not magic bullets, especially if you have insomnia associated with fibromyalgia. For one thing, they can disrupt the body's ability to produce neurochemicals, such as serotonin, which are involved with mood. They are also associated with side effects (see below). Therefore, for effective, safe, long-term relief from insomnia, it is best for you to turn to nondrug methods to aid sleep. Such alternatives are discussed in Chapters 7 and 8.

Specific medications that are helpful for short-term use by some patients with fibromyalgia to help with sleep include the following:

- Low-dose tricyclic antidepressants can help improve deep, restorative sleep.

- Sedatives (hypnotics) such as Ambien (zolpidem), Lunesta (eszopiclone), Rozerem (ramelteon), and Sonata (zaleplon).

- The anticonvulsant drug Lyrica is prescribed for insomnia and fatigue associated with fibromyalgia (see previous discussion on page 79).

- Xyrem, a drug usually prescribed for narcolepsy, has been reported to help promote sleep and relieve pain. See "Did You Know?" under "Analgesics." The most common side effects associated with Xyrem are headache, which may occur in nearly one-quarter of patients; nausea (about 21 percent), and dizziness (about 17 percent). Xyrem is also known as gamma hydroxybutyrate (GHB), or the "date-rape drug."

Side Effects of Sleep Medications

Common side effects associated with use of sleeping pills such as Ambien, Halcion, Lunesta, Rozerem, and Sonata include:

• Burning or tingling in the hands, arms, feet, or legs

• Constipation

• Diarrhea

• Dizziness

• Drowsiness

• Dry mouth or throat

• Gas

• Headache

• Heartburn

• Stomach tenderness or pain

• Uncontrollable tremors

• Unusual dreams or nightmares

• Weakness

Other dangers associated with sleeping pills include un-usual sleep behaviors, called parasomnias. These are behaviors or actions that people engage in while asleep. Parasomnia may include simple sleepwalking as well as sleep eating, making phone calls, driving while asleep, or even having sex while in a sleep state. In 2007, the Food and Drug Administration asked all pharmaceutical manufacturers of sedative-hypnotic drugs to include language on their labels that warns people about the potential risks of taking sleeping pills. Complex sleep behaviors are more likely to occur if you increase your dose, so if you have been prescribed sleeping pills, never take more than your doctor has ordered.

TREATING IRRITABLE BOWEL SYNDROME

If your irritable bowel syndrome (IBS) symptoms are not severe, a nondrug approach, including simple changes in your diet such as increasing fiber intake and eliminating foods that seem to trigger symptoms may be sufficient. Because stress and anxiety can exacerbate irritable bowel symptoms, stress reduction methods are also suggested. These options are discussed in Chapters 7 and 8.

Medical treatment may include OTC laxatives and stool softeners to deal with constipation, although these drugs should not be taken for more than a few days because they can cause dependence. Similarly, OTC medications for diarrhea such as Imodium can be helpful, as can antispasmodic prescription drugs that relieve diarrhea by relaxing muscles in the wall of the gut, as well as reduce cramping that can accompany diarrhea.

One of the often-prescribed antispasmodics for IBS is dicyclomine (Bentyl), which relieves spasms of the muscles of the stomach and intestines by blocking the activity of certain chemicals. This medication can impair your ability to think clearly, as well as cause dry mouth, blurry vision, nausea, and dizziness. You should also be careful not to become overheated when using this drug, because it can reduce your ability to sweat.

A prescription medication for diarrheal IBS is alosetron

hydrochloride (Lotronex), which affects the neurons in the digestive tract to slow the production of waste. Lotronex is indicated only for women who have severe diarrhea-predominant IBS who have not responded adequately to conventional therapy. This drug is associated with infrequent but serious gastrointestinal adverse events, including ischemic colitis and serious complications of constipation that can result in hospitalization and the need for blood transfusions or surgery. Studies show that Lotronex causes constipation in 29 percent of users. Other less common side effects (ones that occur in between 2 and 7 percent of patients) include abdominal pain, gastrointestinal pain, nausea, a distended abdomen, and reflux.

Although it was withdrawn from the market in March 2007, the prescription drug tegaserod maleate (Zelnorm) is still available for "emergency situations" for women who have constipation (not diarrhea) as their main bowel problem as part of severe, chronic IBS. Zelnorm increases the action of serotonin in the intestinal tract. Side effects include gas, back pain, nausea, migraine, dizziness, or joint pain. More serious side effects may include new or worsening stomach pain, blood in the stool, severe stomach pain, ongoing diarrhea, and feeling like you might faint. The drug was withdrawn from the market because patients taking the drug were eight times more likely to suffer a heart attack, stroke, angina, or other cardiovascular complications than people who took a placebo.

GUAIFENESIN THERAPY

Guaifenesin is an ingredient found in many cough syrups that is used to relieve congestion that accompanies the common cold. You may recognize guaifenesin by another name, including Robitussin or Humibid, for example. An endocrinologist and assistant clinical professor at the University of

California, Los Angeles, named Dr. R. Paul St. Amand discovered that this simple cough expectorant can reverse symptoms of fibromyalgia in 90 percent of patients. Dr. St. Amand's interest in fibromyalgia is a personal one, because he has the syndrome as well.

Dr. St. Amand was one of the first scientists to suggest that an excessive amount of phosphate in the body is the cause of fibromyalgia. The theory is that deposits of calcium phosphate accumulate in the muscles, tendons, joints, brain, and other tissues, hindering blood flow, impairing functioning, and resulting in widespread pain and various dysfunctions that are characteristic of fibromyalgia. These deposits are speculated to be caused by an inherited defect in kidney function that prevents the phosphate from being eliminated in urine as it normally is.

Several investigators have looked for evidence of phosphate deposits in fibromyalgia patients, including Muhammad Yunus, MD, of University of Illinois College of Medicine, and Robert Simms, MD, of Boston University. Even the use of NMR spectroscopy did not uncover such deposits. Dr. St. Amand believes they exist.

Because guaifenesin acts on the kidneys to mildly increase the excretion of phosphate, Dr. St. Amand proposed the drug could eliminate phosphate buildup and successfully treat fibromyalgia. Thus he went on to establish a treatment regimen based on this theory, and the treatment includes low doses of guaifenesin.

This approach is controversial, as there seems to be no scientific evidence to support Dr. St. Amand's claims. However, anecdotally some patients have reported they achieved significant improvement on this therapy. A study by researchers at Oregon Health and Science University set out to discover if there was a basis for Dr. St. Amand's claims or the claims of some patients.

At the 1996 Orlando American College of Rheumatology meeting, Robert Bennett, MD, presented his findings on the use of guaifenesin for fibromyalgia in a one-year, placebo-controlled, double-blind (neither patients nor researchers knew what the participants were taking) trial. Twenty female fibromyalgia patients were given 600 mg of guaifenesin twice daily and another 20 were given a placebo for one year. All of the women were told not to take salicylates (e.g., aspirin) because they can interfere with guaifenesin.

Bennett evaluated all the patients every three months and noted their symptoms, tender points, and levels of phosphates and uric acid. None of these factors changed significantly over the year, and the patients' response to guaifenesin was the same as that for the placebo. Proponents of guaifenesin stated that the study was flawed because patients may have used topical products that contain salicylates, but Dr. Bennett explained that evidence of salicylate use would have been seen via elevated uric acid, but this was not observed. He also noted that guaifenesin did not increase the excretion of phosphates—the reason Dr. St. Amand says the therapy works—and so guaifenesin does not appear to be an effective treatment for fibromyalgia.

Despite a lack of evidence that guaifenesin works, some people still turn to it for help. Therefore, you should know that some common side effects associated with guaifenesin treatment include nausea, vomiting, stomach pain, rash, and dizziness. If you take guaifenesin, do not use any topical products while on this therapy, including products that contain aloe, herbs, or salicylates.

INJECTION THERAPIES INVOLVING MEDICATIONS

In addition to taking oral medications, some people with fibromyalgia have specific drugs injected either into a trigger point (trigger point injections) or a nerve (nerve blocks). Both therapies must be performed by a healthcare professional.

Trigger Point Injections

If you have myofascial pain syndrome along with fibromyalgia, a possible treatment option is a trigger point injection. As we noted previously, trigger points are associated with myofascial pain syndrome and are not the same as tender points, which are characteristic of fibromyalgia.

Trigger point injection therapy can relieve the pain and stiffness caused by trigger points, which are like knots or nodules in your muscles. To relieve pain and tenderness, a healthcare professional can inject anesthetics or corticosteroids directly into each trigger point, which provides nearly immediate relief.

A physician can perform trigger point injections in one of two ways, both of which can be done in a doctor's office. Using manual palpation, he or she can locate a trigger point by massaging the skin and then injecting the site. A local anesthetic (usually procaine) is injected, although corticosteroids may be used if the trigger points are especially painful or inflamed.

Another approach is to use needle EMG-guided (electromyography machine) injection, which means the physician uses manual palpation to locate the area of the trigger point. He or she then inserts a needle that sends back information to a monitor, which then allows the doctor to guide the needle directly into the trigger point to place the injected medication. This is the more accurate of the two methods. For both approaches, no more than four trigger points are typically treated at each session.

Even though trigger point injections are designed to relieve myofascial pain syndrome, they can also provide significant relief for people with fibromyalgia. Benefits of trigger point injection are:

• Injections provide quick, long-lasting relief from trigger point pain.

- The amount of referred pain is reduced.

- Injections help to minimize the impact of other symptoms, such as stiffness and fatigue.

- Injections can be done in a doctor's office or at a pain clinic.

Trigger point injections cause some discomfort, and if the points are especially sensitive, you may feel a few seconds of pain when the needle enters the point. Your doctor can administer a sedative before the procedure to numb the area. Side effects of trigger point injections are minimal and may include lightheadedness, tingling, or burning as the anesthetic begins to work, and pain or bruising around the injection site. After the injections, it is best to participate in physical therapy or massage, because stretching the muscles can enhance the benefits of the injections.

Nerve Blocks

A nerve block is an injection inside or around a group of nerve cells that helps to stop regional pain in the body. Nerve blocks, also known as nerve root blocks, provide immediate pain relief. If you have given birth and had an epidural injection, then you have experienced a nerve block injection.

A nerve block works by preventing pain messages from traveling to the brain. The injection can be administered into the spine, which can reduce lower back or leg pain; or injected outside the spinal cord, which can address head, chest, and pelvic pain. Nerve blocks are done by anesthesiologists, who are trained to administer anesthetic drugs via injection.

Medications typically used include anesthetics, corticosteroids, or opioids. Along with immediate relief from pain, a nerve block can also desensitize the nerve, which can provide some future pain relief, as well as a reduction in inflammation. For fibromyalgia patients, nerve blocks can reduce joint and muscle pain, increase range of motion, and thus make exercise, physical therapy, and daily tasks much easier. Side effects are rare, and may include a rash or pain around the injection site, loss of sensation, nausea, vomiting, and nerve damage.

Nerve blocks can be effective when they are combined with other therapies, including exercise, physical therapy, and medications. Because a nerve block provides only temporary relief, you will need to return for another injection every few months, depending on the medication used.

THE BOTTOM LINE

A wide range of OTC and prescription medications taken orally or by injection are available for treatment of fibromyalgia. Given the multifaceted nature of the syndrome, a multitreatment approach is encouraged, and one of the most basic and essential treatments that can be used along with medication is physical exercise. That's our next stop.

CHAPTER SIX

Exercise and Movement Therapies

If the mere mention or thought of exercise makes you want to turn to another chapter, we hope you'll reconsider for a moment. Although your muscles and joints probably already hurt, exercise actually helps to strengthen your muscles, eases joint pain, prevents further injuries, and eventually, it will reduce your pain symptoms as well. It can even make it easier for you to sleep. In fact, avoiding exercise is a huge mistake if you have fibromyalgia.

It may be difficult to take that first step, but once you do, you will discover that the benefits of exercise—physical and emotional—are worth the effort. At one time, doctors thought exercise might make symptoms of fibromyalgia worse or accelerate the disease, so they encouraged their patients to rest. Now, however, research shows that regular exercise, like the type we discuss in this chapter, can keep you fit, reduce pain, improve flexibility, control your weight, improve your ability to sleep, reduce stress and depression, and ultimately give you some control over your fibromyalgia and its symptoms. Some of the benefits come from the fact that exercise helps to restore the body's neurochemical balance and boosts levels of natural painkillers called endorphins. Exercise also gradually strengthens muscles and tones the body, which also helps to control pain. With all of these great benefits, what are you waiting for?

Naturally, we want you to be safe when you begin an exercise program or routine, so you should consult your physician before you begin. He or she may suggest you work with a physical therapist for several sessions so you can determine the most effective and enjoyable physical activities for you.

In this chapter we explore some exercise and movement therapy options for you to consider and to discuss with your healthcare provider. Variety is the spice of life, and so it can be with your exercise choices as well. If you select several options, you can then have an activity to match how you feel on a particular day. Let's get started!

MOVING WITH FIBROMYALGIA

What should your exercise routine or program look like? Since no two people with fibromyalgia are alike, there is no cookie-cutter, one-size-fits-all exercise program. There are, however, some basic elements that should be included in any exercise plan: stretching, aerobics, and strength building. How you choose to accomplish each of these goals is up to you and your healthcare provider.

Stretching

Stretching every day is an essential part of your treatment to help prevent your muscles from becoming stiff and weak. But they are already stiff and weak, you say? Then stretching will gradually revive them and restore flexibility and motion. One great thing about stretching is that you can do it just about anywhere, anytime, and it doesn't require any equipment or cost. What a bargain! Whether you do some simple stretching exercises like the ones mentioned below or those given to you by a physical therapist, doing them every day will help improve your range of motion, keep your muscles supple, and increase your comfort level. If you want to "shake it up" a bit, you might try yoga or pilates or tai

STRETCHES FOR FIBROMYALGIA

Note: Consult your healthcare provider before doing any new exercises.

Quad Stretch. Stand next to a wall and support yourself with one arm. Bend your left knee and bring your heel up to meet your buttocks. You should feel a stretch in the front part of your thigh. Hold, then put your foot back on the floor. Repeat with the other leg. Begin with two or three stretches for each leg.

Calf Stretch. Face a wall and put your hands on the wall for support. Place one leg about one foot length behind the other and press your heel down on the floor. Lean forward toward the wall until you begin to feel a slight stretch in your calf. Hold, then relax. Repeat several times, then do the same stretch with the other leg.

Lower Back and Hip Stretch. Lie flat on the floor on something soft, like a yoga mat or thick towel. Place your hands behind your head and bend your legs so both feet are flat on the floor. Lift your right leg and place the outside of your right heel flat against your left knee, so your right knee is pointing to your right and your right foot is pointing straight up. You should feel a stretch in your lower back and hip. Hold, then release and place your right foot back on the floor. Repeat several times, then do the same with your left leg.

chi, all of which also involve stretching (see details on all three below).

When you begin a stretching routine, do it slowly. Begin with only a few stretches per day and do not hold the stretch for longer than three seconds. You should also hold a stretch only to the point of tightness, never to the point where you feel pain. Over time, you can work up to 10 repetitions of each stretching exercise, extend the amount of time you hold the stretch, and do the stretches two to three times a day.

Aerobics

Aerobics are an important element in fibromyalgia treatment because it improves blood circulation to all parts of the body and strengthens the heart and other muscles. Participating in aerobics prompts the body to produce natural painkillers called endorphins, and these natural substances can help to reduce the stress and strain in your muscles and improve your mood as well.

The goal is not to "pound the pavement" but to enjoy low-impact aerobics, like walking, cycling, dancing, and water aerobics. Begin slowly, especially if you have not exercised in a while. Aim to exercise for 10 minutes three to four times a week at the beginning, and gradually increase each session until you can do 20 to 30 minutes each time. Do aerobic exercise every other day, and on your days off, don't forget to still stretch! On the days you do not do aerobics, you can work on your strength exercises, which we discuss next.

Strength Exercises

Strength exercises are not just for bodybuilders. In fact, a few sessions of light strength training every week is one of the best things you can do when you have fibromyalgia, because strength conditioning can increase your tolerance to pain, improve your range of motion, and help your muscles work more efficiently and comfortably. It's amazing what a few light hand weights can do for you!

You do not need anything fancy or expensive: hand weights that weigh as little as one or two pounds each are a good start. Discuss some possible exercises with a physical therapist or your healthcare provider. Begin with a few exercises and gradually increase the number that you do and the number of sets and repetitions. You could begin, for example, with arm curls and do one set of four repetitions and over a few weeks, increase to three sets of 10 repetitions.

An alternative to weights is an elastic stretchy exercise band. These bands can be purchased in sporting goods stores, online, and from fitness centers. They are convenient and can be taken with you wherever you go without having to deal with carrying extra pounds of weights. Stretchy bands have the same effect on your muscles as hand weights do, but with less strain.

Pilates

Pilates, like yoga, is a therapeutic form of exercise that can significantly reduce various symptoms of fibromyalgia, including pain. But Pilates is more than exercise: it also incorporates relaxation, concentration, breathing, and body alignment, which makes it a holistic movement therapy. Even before you begin to do the exercises, a Pilates instructor should explain each of these four key elements:

- **Relax.** You need to learn how to release the tension and stress in your body so you do not use the wrong muscles when you begin to move.

- **Concentrate.** Pilates involves concentrating on each movement and being aware of your body and how you move each part of it.

- **Align.** It is important to recognize when your body is aligned correctly because proper alignment restores muscle balance and allows your body to move naturally and hopefully with less pain.

- **Breathe.** Proper breathing is essential for any exercise program, and in Pilates the timing of breathing is critical. To gain the maximum benefit from Pilates, you should move when you exhale, which allows you to relax into the stretch.

As you master these four skills, you will begin to learn the movements, which are low-impact, nonaerobic routines that combine stretching and strengthening exercises designed to stabilize your core—abdomen, back, and pelvic floor muscles. This creates a strong base that best supports the body, improves posture, reduces muscle tension and joint pain, improves coordination and overall muscle tone, and promotes relaxation. It can alleviate stress incontinence and fatigue, and also help reduce fibrofog and anxiety.

A pilot study of Pilates in fibromyalgia patients was conducted in 2009. Fifty women were assigned to either a Pilates exercise program of one hour three times a week for 12 weeks, or to a home exercise program of relaxation and stretching. After 12 weeks, women in the Pilates groups reported significant improvement in pain, functional abilities, and quality of life compared with the control group. By week 24, however, there was no difference in improvement between the two groups. This study gives us two bits of information. One is that Pilates can provide great improvement in a shorter time than can a home exercise program of relaxation and stretching, and the other is that Pilates is an effective optional exercise routine.

You may have heard that the Pilates method uses more than 500 types of controlled exercises, but you certainly do not have to learn all of them! You will work closely with your Pilates instructor to choose the movements that are best suited for your needs and goals.

Yoga

Yoga is a mentally relaxing, physically invigorating form of body and mind exercise that has helped many people who have fibromyalgia. "Practicing yoga makes my body feel alive, and it hurts less," says Monica, a forty-five-year-old mother of two who has had fibromyalgia for about five years. "The gentle stretching is perfect. I do as much as I can, and I always feel like I've accomplished something when I'm done. I practice a little each day, and when I miss a day I notice the difference."

More than 15 million American practice yoga on a regular basis, and you can be one of them. As little as 10 minutes a day can help you improve strength, increase endurance, and achieve a sense of mental relaxation. People with fibromyalgia who practice yoga report being able to sleep better, have greater endurance, feel less tension and stress, and have improved concentration. Yoga is perfect for beginners: all you need is enough space to move around, a large soft towel or yoga mat to place on the floor, and the desire to learn and heal.

Yoga incorporates three main activities that integrate mind, body, and spirit.

- **Postures (asanas).** Postures in yoga are gentle stretches that you hold for a short time. There are hundreds of different postures, and so you are guaranteed to find some that fit your physical abilities. Although yoga postures are done using slow, gentle movements, they are powerful and can improve circulation, enhance flexibility, relieve tension, and strengthen your muscles.

- **Breathing (pranayama).** Deep breathing exercises are done in sync with the postures. It helps to have a professional yoga instructor show you how to breathe correctly and to integrate the breathing with your movements. Yoga breathing is forced and calculated and is designed to increase the flow of oxygen and nutrients in the body. Proper breathing during yoga is important because there is a direct connection between how you breathe and the amount of tension in your body. When you are under stress, your muscles tighten and your breathing becomes shallow. Shallow breathing does not deliver enough oxygen to your cells and can contribute to more tension in your muscles, and thus result in more pain. Therefore breathing is an essential part of the yoga experience.

- **Meditation (dhyana).** The third element is meditation, which completes the complete yoga experience. While you practice yoga, you are encouraged to let tension and worries disappear. Entering into a meditative state is the way those who practice yoga achieve this. Again, an instructor can help you learn how to meditate while also doing the postures and breathing exercises.

Before you go running to your nearest yoga center, it is good to know about the different types of yoga. Depending on your physical abilities and needs, one type of yoga may be more beneficial for you than another. Some forms of yoga, such as bikram yoga and ashtanga yoga, are physically challenging and typically recommended for individuals who are athletic. Other forms are more conducive for people with fibromyalgia.

- **Hatha yoga.** This form of yoga is among the most popular and commonly practiced forms in the United States. It is often recommended for people who have fibromyalgia and arthritis because you are encouraged to perform the postures at your own pace. Hatha yoga is a slow and mellow form of the practice and a form that makes it easier to integrate the breathing and meditation into the entire routine.

- **Viniyoga.** This form is popular among people who live with chronic pain, older adults, and people who are recovering from injuries. It is a slow, individualized type of yoga that focuses on helping you improve balance, coordination, and strength.

If you do decide to try yoga, look for an instructor who has worked with people who have fibromyalgia and/or arthritis, as they are more likely to know which postures to suggest and how to help you through them. Classes are offered at private yoga centers, community centers, and health clubs. Once you have learned the postures, breathing, and meditation, you can do the practice in the comfort of your home without an instructor. At any time you can add to or change your routine. Yoga is a movement therapy that you can tailor to your own personal needs, energy, and physical fitness level.

"Yoga is something I never imagined myself doing," says Justin, who was diagnosed with fibromyalgia three years ago. "Now here I am, at 46 and learning new ways to stretch and move my body. Fibromyalgia has made it so difficult to move much of the time, but yoga keeps me going."

Tai Chi

Slow, gentle, and easy: that's how you do tai chi, a practice that was originally developed thousands of years ago as a martial art. Today tai chi is a form of exercise that is often described as "poetry in motion" and "movement meditation." Tai chi is a low-impact form of movement that is kind to the body's joints and muscles, yet it is deceptively power-

YOGA TIPS

- Never stretch to a point that causes pain. If you begin to feel pain, stop or ease up on your stretch.

- Begin with just five minutes of practice a day, and gradually increase your sessions to 25 or 30 minutes.

- Take a class. We realize that most yoga classes last for at least 45 minutes, and maybe as long as an hour or more, which is much longer than you should do yoga as a beginner, and especially as a person who has fibromyalgia. Look for a class that may cater to people who have health issues, and/or a beginners' class that may be offered for a shorter amount of time. Remember, you do not have to participate in the entire class. Talk to the instructor and explain what you wish to learn and your limitations. You may also be able to find a yoga class at a hospital or clinic that is specifically for people who have medical conditions.

- Remember to breathe and meditate. It will take time for you to become comfortable combining postures, breathing, and meditation, so do not get frustrated. It all comes with practice.

ful, because the slow movements gradually build muscle strength, reduce widespread pain and joint stiffness, relieve stress and anxiety, improve quality of sleep, increase mental clarity (decrease fibrofog), and improve mood. Thus it works on the body, mind, and spirit all at once.

Tai chi is an excellent movement therapy for fibromyalgia

patients because it is gentle, it allows you to do only what you are capable of doing, it can provide many benefits, and it is a holistic therapy that encompasses mind, body, and spirit. Although you may be able to learn tai chi from a video or DVD, attending classes is the best way to experience it. Due to the increasing popularity of tai chi, many cities and towns have classes that are available through community and senior centers and health facilities, including hospitals and clinics. Let the instructor know you have fibromyalgia, and, if possible, find one who is familiar with the syndrome.

MOTIVATIONAL TIPS

- **Set reasonable goals.** If your goal is to walk 30 minutes every other day, begin by walking five minutes. When that feels good, then increase it to eight or 10 minutes each session. Make gradual, comfortable progress toward your goals, and you will not get discouraged.

- **Start slow and easy.** This is important for everyone, but especially if you have not exercised in a while or at all. Pushing too hard at the beginning may result in strained, sprained, or otherwise injured muscles or joints, and we don't want that to happen!

- **Keep a record of your progress.** One way is to set a goal, say, "I want to walk to the beach" (and you live 100 miles from the nearest beach). If you walk about three miles per hour, that's 20 minutes per mile, so it would take you 2,000 minutes to walk to the beach. Set up a chart with 2,000 minutes at one end or at the top and track your progress. Every time you walk, subtract your time from 2,000 until you reach the beach!

- **Buddy up!** Exercising seems easier and is more enjoyable when you share the time with a friend. You may want to join an aerobics class or water aerobics class so you can share in a group experience on occasion. It can be much more fun to sweat with others!

- **Plug in!** Listen to music, motivational tapes, books on tape, etc. while you exercise.

- **Change your routine.** Variety can make your exercise sessions more exciting and seem much less like work! Perhaps you can do several different types of aerobics, for example: on alternate days do walking, stationary biking, an aerobics class, water aerobics, dancing. If walking is the only aerobics you can do, change your route, walk through a mall, enroll in a walkathon, walk during lunch—there are many possibilities.

- **If you need to skip a day, do it.** Sometimes you may feel like you just can't walk or ride a bike or lift your weights. That's okay: just be sure to return to your schedule for the rest of the week. We do suggest that even if you skip a day of aerobics and strength exercises, you should do some stretching exercises, because they really will make you feel better.

PHYSICAL THERAPY

Physical therapy, also known as physiotherapy, is a treatment approach that focuses on helping individuals decrease pain, increase physical mobility, and improve quality of life. For people who have fibromyalgia, physical therapy can make a significant positive impact on many aspects of their daily life.

A physical therapist (or physiotherapist) can evaluate your physical capabilities, identify your specific treatment needs, and then show you various exercises and routines you can do at home based on your unique situation that will help you improve muscle strength, joint function, and overall mobility.

During your first visit with a physical therapist, she or he will assess your current physical state, ask you if you have been doing any type of physical exercise or therapies, if you have any sleep problems, what your anxiety or stress level is and what you hope to achieve through physical therapy. You will be asked questions about your medical history and then undergo a physical exam that will include an evaluation of your gait, posture, muscle strength, reflexes, joint flexibility, and range of motion.

Once the assessment is done, you and the therapist can develop a treatment plan that suits your needs. The plan can be as simple or as complex as you want, taking into consideration any time, cost, and physical limitations. The physical therapist can devise a stretching, strength, and aerobics program for you, as well as suggest or offer different types of treatments, which could include the following:

- **Manual treatments.** These may include different types of massage and stretching exercises that can help increase range of motion and reduce swelling and pain. Massage is discussed in detail in Chapter 7.

- **Physical treatments.** Commonly used physical treatments include water therapy such as whirlpool or the use of deep heating with hot packs or paraffin waxing. These approaches can increase muscle and joint flexibility and decrease swelling.

- **Aquatic treatments.** The buoyancy of water can allow you to do low-impact exercises without placing strain and stress on your muscles and joints. Many people with fibromyalgia find they can do exercises in the water that they cannot do out of the water. Not only can aquatic exercises improve your physical well-being and reduce symptoms, they can also make you feel better emotionally, giving you a feeling of accomplishment. One form of aquatic therapy called Watsu (see below) has been shown to be especially beneficial for people who have fibromyalgia and various forms of arthritis.

- **Electrotherapy treatments.** Types of electrotherapy treatments include neurofeedback and electrical muscle stimulation. These therapies can promote healing and decrease pain and muscle spasms. Neurofeedback is discussed in Chapter 7.

- **Trigger point injections.** Many physical therapists are trained to give trigger point injections. These treatments deliver anesthetics or corticosteroids into specific painful points and provide rapid relief. Trigger point injections are discussed in Chapter 5.

Watsu

Do you want to watsu? If you have never heard of watsu, you may be surprised to learn that there are watsu practitioners in more than 40 countries, including the United States. Watsu is a combination of "water" and "shiatsu" and is a form of water therapy (hydrotherapy). Through the integration of buoyancy, warm water, massage, and water resistance, people with fibromyalgia who participate in watsu can enjoy an improvement in their symptoms.

Advocates of watsu report that after just one session, you will experience increased range of motion and muscle relaxation, and decreased pain and muscle spasms. The longer term benefits include improved sleep patterns, better digestion, greater decreases in pain, reduced anxiety, and improved immune system response. Several small studies of people with fibromyalgia and of those with chronic pain support these claims.

You may enjoy these benefits as well if you try watsu. Here's what you might expect from a watsu session, although practitioners insist there is no "typical" session—each experience is tailor-made for you. One common factor is that practitioners always ask clients if they have any fear of water, what they want from the sessions, and if there are any physical conditions that require attention. Once you step into the warm pool of water, you place yourself in the hands—and arms—of the practitioner. You will lie back in the water, supported by the therapist. Sometimes you will be in a cradling position similar to a fetus in the womb; other times you will stretch out in the water. Throughout the entire session, the therapist will isolate your muscles and stretch them to improve flexibility and reduce tension.

Watsu is both a physical and an emotional experience: it is about letting go, physically and emotionally, and allowing someone to hold and support you and feeling your own lightness in the water. For some people, it takes several sessions before they can relax enough to allow the practitioner to perform the stretches and massages without feeling tense.

While you are in the water and your body is being stretched, you also pay attention to your breathing. Watsu includes the

Water Breath Dance, in which you float in the arms of the practitioner, who lets you sink slightly as you breathe out and let the water lift you as you breathe in. When this cycle is repeated again and again, it creates a connection with the stretches and moves your body makes in the water.

If you are interested in trying watsu, practitioners can be found through the Worldwide Aquatic Bodywork Association (see "Resources").

PAULA: AN EXERCISE SUCCESS STORY

Paula was a 26-year-old graduate student when she was diagnosed with fibromyalgia. She had always been active, participating in field hockey and track in high school, and still running once she entered college. During her second and last year of graduate school, she began experiencing extreme fatigue, widespread pain, and symptoms of irritable bowel syndrome. At first she explained it away as working too hard on her studies and at a part-time job as a waitress. After several months, however, it became obvious that something else was wrong.

"I could barely get out of bed in the morning to go to class, and I had to quit my job," she said. "I began to worry that I wouldn't even be able to finish my course work. I certainly wasn't able to run anymore, I wasn't sleeping well, and I was having trouble concentrating." After consulting several doctors, she finally was referred to a rheumatologist, who diagnosed fibromyalgia. Although Paula was happy to get a diagnosis, she became anxious when she began investigating her treatment options.

"I didn't want to take drugs, yet I also didn't want to be in pain all the time. Since I was so used to being physically active, I was encouraged when the rheumatologist recommended I go to a physical therapist who could work with me."

While Paula did agree to take an analgesic, she was

determined to fight the fibromyalgia with exercise. "I read some studies about the benefits of exercise, and that made sense to me, even though I didn't feel like I could do much of anything. But I had been physical enough in the past to know that a good exercise routine was well worth a shot."

Paula and her physical therapist began with easy stretching and strength-building exercises, and gradually she tried other activities. "I found that tai chi was helpful because it is gentle yet good for strength and balance," she said. "I also got bored with the stretching exercises, so I joined a beginners' yoga class and learned enough to do it at home several times a week." Within just two months of starting her various exercise routines, Paula says she felt much better.

"I still have good and bad days," she says, "but the good days are outnumbering the bad ones. On bad days I just do some easy stretching or some water aerobics, which I just started a few weeks ago, but on the good ones I can do more. The exercise has allowed me to really minimize the amount of painkillers I take, and it also seems to help me sleep better. I'm also taking probiotics for my bowel symptoms, and I watch my diet, too. I'm convinced that people can take charge of their fibromyalgia instead of having it take charge of them if they stay active and are willing to try different things."

THE BOTTOM LINE

The old adage is "energy begets energy," and it is true in fibromyalgia in the fight against fatigue. Movement and exercise also benefit the other key symptom of the syndrome: pain. Regular physical activity is critical for fibromyalgia patients, and we hope you can embrace this challenge, because in the long run, it is probably the best therapy you can do.

CHAPTER SEVEN

Alternative Mind/Body Therapies

Along with nutritional and herbal supplements, some fibromyalgia patients turn to other alternative and complementary therapy options that help relieve symptoms and heal the body and mind in different ways. More and more conventional physicians are practicing what is called integrative or complementary medicine, introducing or recommending mind/body techniques to their patients. This is an especially critical and beneficial step for people who have fibromyalgia, since it is such a challenge to treat.

If your search for an effective treatment is hitting a few hurdles or if you are ready to try something different that has been shown to be effective and safe in people who have symptoms associated with fibromyalgia, then read on. You will find a wealth of options in this chapter. But do not feel overwhelmed by the choices! We suggest you read through them, then choose one or two that fit your symptoms and sound like something you would like to try. We hope you will find one or more mind/body therapies that bring you relief and an improved quality of life.

ACUPUNCTURE AND ACUPRESSURE

Acupuncture and acupressure have become increasingly popular in the United States. These millennia-old Chinese practices can be especially effective in reducing certain symptoms of fibromyalgia that involve pain, including chronic muscle pain, tension headache, and migraine, and in easing symptoms of gastrointestinal problems. Both acupuncture and acupressure work by restoring balance to the body, which results in an improvement in overall function and can also treat specific symptoms.

Acupuncture

Acupuncture uses very thin, metallic needles to stimulate special sites called acupoints throughout the body. Practitioners explain that inserting these needles helps release or enhance the flow of the life force energy, or chi (qi), through the body, which in turn alleviates symptoms such as pain.

Scientists believe the pain-relieving benefits may occur because stimulating these acupoints may block pain signals from reaching the brain and increase the level of the body's natural painkillers called endorphins. Specifically, acupuncture appears to increase levels of certain brain chemicals (e.g., serotonin, beta-endorphin, endomorphin-1), all of which help to reduce pain symptoms.

Acupuncture professionals know which points to treat to address the areas that are causing your pain or imbalance. Acupuncture treatments are painless, although the thought of being stuck with needles does not appeal to everyone. Typically acupuncture treatments are given over a period of two to three months, with a total of six to 12 treatments, depending on your unique situation.

Acupressure

If needles are not your cup of tea, then you might consider acupressure. Acupressure is similar to acupuncture in that the same acupoints are treated, but no needles are involved. Instead, practitioners apply pressure to the acupoints using their fingers, knuckles, elbows, palms, or feet. Typically the pressure is held for three to 10 seconds. One advantage of acupressure over acupuncture is that you or a spouse, friend, or family member can learn which acupoints to treat and you can do it yourself. For best results, however, consult a professional for the proper treatment sites.

Acupuncture and Acupressure for Fibromyalgia

Can acupuncture and acupressure really help? Research supports the claims, as do the many fibromyalgia patients who turn to these Chinese therapies. In a study conducted by the Mayo Clinic, for example, 50 patients were assigned to one of two groups: one group received actual acupuncture treatments while the other group was given simulated acupuncture. Both groups participated in six sessions over a two- to three-week period.

The patients who received the real acupuncture said they had improvements in fatigue and anxiety. Most of the participants said they enjoyed the treatments. Side effects were minimal and included bruising and soreness among those who received the actual treatments. Overall, patients who received acupuncture experienced relief that was equal to what they achieved when taking medications. The benefits of acupuncture seem to last for up to one month beyond the last treatment received.

If acupuncture or acupressure seems like something you would like to try, this is what a typical first session may be like. The therapist will discuss your medical history with you and talk about your general health, your fibromyalgia symptoms, and what you would like to achieve with treatment. He or she will also ask about any other treatments you are receiving or what you have tried in the past and about your experience with the treatment.

The therapist will then check three pulse points in each wrist, note the color of your face, and evaluate the color and texture of your tongue. This information helps the practitioner determine which acupoints should be treated. Usually six to 12 acupoints are treated during a single session, and no more than 15 acupoints.

Some acupuncture therapists use variations on traditional acupuncture techniques. One is called moxibustion, in which the therapist heats the needles with dried herb sticks to activate and warm the acupoint. Another is electroacupuncture, in which a very mild electrical current is delivered through a few acupuncture needles. The treatments usually last 10 to 20 minutes and are most helpful for people who have chronic pain, which is the main reason this approach can benefit people who have fibromyalgia.

Every person reacts differently to acupuncture and acupressure treatments. First of all, you should not experience any pain, although you may feel some tingling or aching at each acupoint. After a session, some people feel invigorated, while others feel very relaxed (and sleepy if they have been having sleep problems). You might feel a heaviness in your legs and arms. Side effects are rare, but people have been known to faint, experience headache or fatigue, or feel a little nauseous. These symptoms are temporary and are actually an indication that the practitioner has stimulated the healing process.

BIOFEEDBACK

This alternative treatment approach operates on the idea that you can reduce your fibromyalgia symptoms by learning how the power of your mind can influence your body's responses. This therapy was originally designed to treat a variety of conditions, including chronic pain, fatigue, and paralysis, and it has helped many people reduce various symptoms of the syndrome.

The process of biofeedback involves being "hooked up" to a machine—via painless electrodes attached to your skin—that records electric impulses sent out by your body in the form of muscle twitches, brain waves, or temperature. The machine then "feeds back" the signals to you in the form of beeps or lights, which are shown on the biofeedback screen. If the machine detects that your muscles are twitching fast, for example, the machine will send out rapid beeps. This is also an indication that your body is under stress. Your goal is to find a way to reduce the number of beeps, which in turn will relax your body's electrical impulses and therefore reduce your symptoms.

After a series of biofeedback sessions, you will learn how to recognize your body's reactions to stress and become more attuned to your body's needs. At that point, you may be able to do biofeedback at home, without the machine. There are, however, biofeedback devices you can purchase for home use.

There are several types of biofeedback. Your biofeedback therapist may try several of them together to help you achieve your goals.

- **Electromyograph.** This is the most common type of biofeedback and the one in which the device measures the electricity that your muscles emit. This type is especially helpful for fibromyalgia patients to reduce muscle pain and stiffness.

- **Electroderm.** A device monitors the sweating reflex, and it is used to treat depression and anxiety.

- **Brainwave electroencephalogram.** This device measures your brain waves and is helpful in correcting depression, sleep disturbances, and other similar ailments.

• **Breathing.** This form gives you information about your breathing and pulse rates. It is used to treat fatigue and anxiety.

Another form of biofeedback, called neurofeedback, uses a different approach and is covered in a separate entry in this chapter.

When we look at the research, one study that used electromyograph biofeedback in people with fibromyalgia reported that patients experienced significant improvement in pain reduction, tender points, and psychologically. In another study, fibromyalgia patients who participated in 15 biofeedback sessions reported a reduction in the number of tender points and an improvement in pain and muscle stiffness. These benefits lasted for up to six months.

What can biofeedback do for you? If you are interested in learning more, your healthcare provider may be able to provide you with a referral. Biofeedback is usually practiced by licensed professionals and is used by psychologists, physical therapists, and psychiatrists. See "Resources" for biofeedback associations.

CHIROPRACTIC CARE

Chiropractic care is based on the theory that the body is a connected system that depends on your bones, muscles, joints, tendons, and ligaments to keep it functioning. Pain, illness, and disability are caused by misalignments of the skeleton system, but they can be treated and corrected by restoring balance to the system.

Many mainstream medical professionals have accepted chiropractic care as an effective treatment for a wide variety of ailments. One of those conditions is fibromyalgia. A chiropractor uses different techniques, including stretches, manipulations, and adjustments to the spine to restore balance and alignment to the body, which in turn can reduce or eliminate pain symptoms.

One reason chiropractic treatment is beneficial is because many people with fibromyalgia have many tender points all over their body, resulting in back pain, neck pain, and pain in the extremities. A chiropractor can perform some simple adjustments to the neck and spine to restore alignment, and in the process pain is often reduced.

Not all chiropractors are the same, however. There are two main techniques that chiropractors can practice:

- Straight chiropractors follow the original teachings of chiropractic medicine and focus their work on manipulations to restore alignment and relieve pain.

- Mixed chiropractors combine the original teachings and techniques of adjustment and manipulation with diet, massage, and exercise. Most chiropractors fall into this category.

Chiropractors can help you if you have cervical spinal stenosis, a condition that affects many people who have fibromyalgia. Cervical spinal stenosis is a condition in which the coverings of the upper spine, called the meninges, become compressed, causing severe pain that can affect the entire body. Chiropractors can make adjustments to the head and neck to relieve the compression, which help to reduce or eliminate the pain.

Several studies have explored the benefits of chiropractic care in fibromyalgia patients and results suggest that chiropractic care can benefit some patients by reducing pain and improving sleep. If you decide to try chiropractic care, consult your healthcare provider who is managing your fibromyalgia to make sure chiropractic care is a safe treatment for you. Although rare, chiropractic manipulations of the neck and spine have been associated with an increased risk of heart attack and stroke. People who have osteoporosis have an increased risk of bone fractures associated with manipulations.

Make sure you choose a practitioner who is used to working with people who have fibromyalgia. Most people have to attend several sessions before they experience noticeable relief. You can get a referral to a chiropractor from your healthcare provider or you can contact a chiropractic organization (see "Resources") for a list of licensed practitioners in your area.

COGNITIVE BEHAVIORAL THERAPY

Therapists everywhere are finding great success with this psychotherapy approach for their patients, and among their success stories are people who have fibromyalgia. Cognitive behavioral therapy is a combination of cognitive therapy and behavioral therapy, and it emphasizes the importance of thinking how you feel and what you do. In cognitive therapy you work to change or eliminate the impact that your thought patterns have on your symptoms, while in behavioral therapy you work to change behaviors that may contribute to your symptoms.

Here's how cognitive behavioral therapy can help fibromyalgia. The pain, fatigue, and other symptoms of fibromyalgia are often worsened by feelings of stress, hopelessness, and other negative emotions. Cognitive behavioral therapy can help you to identify those emotions and teach you how to deal with them in a way that will not cause them to flare up. Once you can identify your destructive thoughts, you can learn how to replace them with thoughts that can result in more positive, healing reactions. This therapy can also show you how to change or modify some of your behaviors and actions, which can reduce the severity of your pain and fatigue.

If you decide to try cognitive behavioral therapy, your psychotherapist will discuss your symptoms with you and your thoughts, feelings, and emotions about having to live and deal with fibromyalgia. The goal of your therapy sessions will be to find connections between how you feel about your symptoms and the symptoms themselves, and to find ways to deal with your emotions in ways that will improve the symptoms. The psychotherapist will help you learn how to challenge your negative beliefs, focus on prioritizing activities in your life, and accept that relapses can happen.

Fibromyalgia patients usually attend between six and 20 sessions. In one study, people with fibromyalgia attended eight one-hour sessions, and all of them reported reduced pain, better sleep, and improved fatigue after just eight sessions. Many of the participants also said their mood improved as well. Naturally, the number of sessions any one person needs is highly individual. If you combine cognitive behavioral therapy with other methods, including regular exercise and relaxation methods (e.g., meditation, yoga, biofeedback), it can be even more effective.

Your healthcare provider should be able to refer you to a cognitive behavioral therapist, but you can also check with a national organization for qualified individuals in your area (see "Resources").

FREQUENCY SPECIFIC MICROCURRENT (FSM)

Frequency specific microcurrent (FSM) is an FDA-approved treatment that works by applying electrical stimulation to a patient's muscles via electronic equipment. This therapy was first used in the 1980s in Europe to treat injured athletes, and it has been proven to be a safe, noninvasive treatment for

DID YOU KNOW?

Results of a small study published in June 2010 reported that a form of "mind/body" therapy that focuses on the role emotions play in physical pain may provide some relief to people with fibromyalgia. In the study, 45 women with fibromyalgia either learned a technique called "affective self-awareness" or were on a wait-list for treatment. The treated women learned about the emotion-pain connection and certain techniques, such as mindfulness meditation and "expressive" writing to help them recognize and deal with emotions that may have been contributing to their pain. Six months after the intervention, 46 percent of the women had at least a 30 percent reduction in pain severity, and 21 percent had a 50 percent or greater pain reduction. This was only the first clinical trial to test affective self-awareness for fibromyalgia, so stay tuned for further research results.

fibromyalgia, as well as sports injuries, lupus, irritable bowel syndrome, endometriosis, shingles, and herpes.

During an FSM treatment, the practitioner uses specialized gloves that can detect abnormal electron frequencies in the muscular tissue in a person's body. Once the doctor finds abnormalities in the muscle, a microcurrent is administered to neutralize them.

Studies show that FSM can improve circulation, increase energy, help repair damaged tissues, and detoxify the body. In a study of 160 people with fibromyalgia conducted from 1999 to 2003, patients treated with FSM reported that their pain levels decreased from a high point of 7.3 to a low point of 1.3 after their first treatment. That sounds encouraging!

As with most therapies that detoxify the body, there are some side effects as the body adjusts during the cleansing process. Thus, patients who try FSM may experience nausea, fatigue, temporary pain, and drowsiness. These reactions can be experienced during the treatment itself and for up to 24 hours post-treatment.

To help alleviate side effects, it is helpful to take antioxidants (e.g., vitamins C and E, beta-carotene, selenium) to neutralize the toxins as they are released and to drink two quarts of water after your treatment as well. Yes, that sounds like a lot of water, but drink it slowly. It will wash away the toxins and the side effects associated with the treatment process.

You can find qualified practitioners of FSM in health clinics throughout the United States. It is considered a physical therapy practice, and a well-staffed physical therapy clinic may be your best bet.

HYPNOTHERAPY

All you skeptics, take note: research shows that hypnosis can benefit people who have fibromyalgia. It is not hocus-pocus; in fact, you can learn self-hypnosis from a professional and then do it yourself whenever you need it.

Under the guidance of a well-trained, professional hypnotherapist, you can be given suggestions that work toward your specific goals, such as getting better sleep, exercising more, and reducing pain. When you are in a hypnotic state, you will feel completely relaxed, and you will be able to focus on the goal you have selected. Everyone has their own level of susceptibility to hypnosis, so your success will depend on how easily you can be hypnotized and your ability to hypnotize yourself.

A number of studies show that hypnosis can help individuals reduce chronic pain in general and fibromyalgia symptoms in particular. One study found that hypnosis reduced the number of tender points in patients who were hypnotized over several months, while another, published in the *American Journal of Clinical Hypnosis* reported that psychological treatment produced better symptom relief than conventional medical treatment, especially when hypnosis was included in the treatment process.

Trust is an important issue when you are dealing with hypnosis, so be sure you feel completely comfortable with the hypnotherapist you choose. Once you have had several sessions, you can choose to learn self-hypnosis so you can enjoy the benefits anytime you feel the need. You can ask your healthcare practitioner or local hospital or university for a referral, or contact an organization that specializes in hypnotherapists (see "Resources").

LIGHT THERAPY

Light can be a powerful healing source that has the ability to relieve various types of chronic pain and depression. Also

DID YOU KNOW?

An article that reviewed 13 studies of hypnosis for the treatment of chronic pain found that hypnosis consistently produced significant decreases in pain. Most of the studies involved self-hypnosis. The review, which was conducted by researchers at Texas A&M University College of Medicine, found that hypnosis was generally more effective than nonhypnotic interventions such as physical therapy and education.

known as phototherapy, light therapy delivers colored, low-energy forms of light to different areas of the body to trigger the release of hormones and promote healing.

Light therapy is practiced by physicians, physical therapists, and psychologists and used to treat muscle pain, depression, fatigue, and insomnia in people who have fibromyalgia. This therapy is also used to treat arthritis, migraine, and soft tissue injuries. You can choose from three different types of light therapy: bright light, colored light, and low-level laser.

Bright Light Therapy

Bright light therapy, which is the one most commonly used, is based on the concept that the body is in tune with light. Indeed, our lives are largely regulated by change in natural light. Known as the circadian rhythm, the body's sleep cycle, energy levels, and moods are all in sync with natural light changes. Bright light therapy uses high-powered fluorescent lights to help trigger the release of certain hormones which will then restore the body's natural circadian rhythm and overall health.

Bright light therapy can be done at home if you have a light box, a small box that contains a number of full-spectrum (white) lightbulbs. Perhaps you have heard of using a light box to treat a type of depression called SAD—seasonal affective disorder. Treatment is easy: all you do is sit in front of the box—without looking directly into the light—for anywhere between 15 minutes and three hours, depending on what you are treating. The idea is that your body absorbs the light and impacts your hormones while you read, sew, or do other leisure activities.

Color Light Therapy

Add a little color to your life, and perhaps a lot of relief, with color light therapy. This form of therapy is becoming more popular with people who have chronic pain. Four main colors are usually used in color light therapy: red, blue, violet, and white. When your eyes perceive the light (which is UV filtered), the light energy converts into electric impulses, which travel through your brain and trigger the release of certain hormones, including serotonin (the mood hormone) and endorphins (the body's natural painkillers). Thus, color light therapy can improve mood and reduce pain.

You don't have to look at the colored lights to be treated. The colors can be applied directly to certain areas of your body as well. In either case, color therapy is relaxing and usually lasts between 15 and 60 minutes.

Low Level Laser Therapy

Low level laser therapy involves applying low-frequency laser beams to painful areas of the body. It is also referred to as cold light therapy because the lasers do not produce heat. What they can do, however, is help reduce pain and promote healing which is done by increasing the energy levels of the cells in the body. Using a special laser wand, the healthcare provider focuses the laser beam on a certain part of the body. The light sends out photons that the body's cells absorb. The photons are converted into cellular energy by the cells, which boosts the body's ability to heal and thus eliminates pain. Treatments typically last about 15 to 20 minutes and provide immediate relief.

Have you seen the light? Many fibromyalgia patients have, and they are reporting success. In a study of low-energy laser therapy in 40 women with fibromyalgia, half of the women were treated daily for two weeks (except for weekends) while the other half got placebo laser treatment. At the end of the study, the women who had received the laser therapy reported a significant improvement in pain, muscle spasm, morning stiffness, and the total number of tender points when compared with the placebo group.

The only side effects reported with light therapy are eye

sensitivity and irritation, and mild nausea at the beginning of the sessions, which goes away. Some patients become restless or overstimulated by light therapy, in which case your therapist (or you) can reduce the amount of time you get treated. If you have glaucoma, cataracts, or other eye diseases, or if you have epilepsy, skin sensitivities, or bipolar disorder, talk to your healthcare provider before trying any form of light therapy.

MASSAGE

Who doesn't like a massage? Touch is one of the strongest healing forces we have, and massage therapy is an effective way to transmit relief and healing through carefully applied touch. A massage therapist, or perhaps your spouse, friend, or family member who has been shown some simple strokes, can manipulate your muscles and soft tissues to relieve stress, reduce pain, and increase flexibility. Although massage is typically done with the hands, special instruments or devices also can be utilized to work the tension out of tense muscles. You or a therapist can also use hot and cold therapies as part of the massage to enhance blood flow and relax muscles.

No one is exactly certain what goes on underneath those massaging fingers that makes this therapy so helpful. Scientists believe massage enhances the production of certain pain blockers, such as endorphins, norepinephrine, and serotonin. These hormones can counteract pain messages that are transmitted by the brain. Whatever the reason, massage is one of the most beneficial treatments for relieving the pain and fatigue associated with fibromyalgia.

Types of Massage

If you are interested in massage, you have a wide variety of types from which to choose. Several are relatively easy for

DID YOU KNOW?

Benefits of massage therapy for fibromyalgia patients include reduced pain, less stiffness, improved sleep, decreased stress and depression, improved range of motion, increased flexibility, and enhanced blood circulation to the muscles. In one study, people with fibromyalgia who enjoyed 10 30-minute massage sessions reported a 38 percent decrease in pain symptoms and a significant improvement in sleep problems.

your spouse or family member to learn, while others are best enjoyed by a professional massage therapist. Here are a few types of massage that are beneficial for relieving fibromyalgia symptoms.

- **Swedish massage.** One of the most popular forms of massage in the United States. It is designed to increase the amount of oxygen delivered to the muscles, which improves flexibility and helps to eliminate toxins from the body. People who perform Swedish massage usually use long, gliding massage movements with their thumbs, fingertips, and palms. They can also include kneading and tapping techniques. Although a Swedish massage from a professional is ideal, an option is for a partner or friend to learn a few simple techniques and give you a massage.

- **Deep tissue massage.** A vigorous therapy in which the practitioner attempts to loosen areas of inflexible muscles and tissues, deep tissue massage uses deep, pressurized strokes that target the deep layers of your tendons and muscles. The strokes are slower and deeper than in Swedish massage, and you may feel some pain after your treatment session. Although the pain typically disappears within a day or two of treatment, this form of massage is not for everyone who has fibromyalgia.

- **Myofascial release.** This form of massage focuses on your body's fascia, that thin layer of tissue that covers your muscles and organs. In fibromyalgia, the fascia frequently become short and tense, causing pain. Myofascial release therapy incorporates stretching techniques that can reduce the pull of the connective tissue on the bones, which allows the muscles to relax and lengthen and the organs to expand. The result is a reduction in pain.

- **Reflexology.** This form of massage involves pressing and massaging certain reflex areas on the feet and hands that correspond with all of the areas of the body and the organs. When these areas are pressed and massaged, they encourage the body to naturally restore its own balance. With reflexology, you or your partner or friend can learn enough so you can use this therapy at home. Of course, having a professional reflexologist do the job is a big plus, but it's good to know that there is something you can learn and do yourself, allowing you to take your healing into your own hands, literally!

When looking for a massage therapist, it is critical to find one who knows how to work with people who have fibromyalgia. This is especially important if you are experiencing a flare-up of your symptoms. During a flare-up, an insufficient amount of oxygen may be contributing to your pain. Because

DID YOU KNOW?

If you have a massage school in your area, contact them about their student rates. Student massage therapists need people to practice on, and the schools typically offer discounted massage sessions—sometimes even free ones—to the public. These sessions are supervised by a professional massage therapist, but the massage is performed by the student. Make sure you let them know you have fibromyalgia! A massage school is also a great place to look for a professional massage therapist.

massage increases oxygen delivery to the muscles, a massage may be just what your body needs during a flare-up. However, you may need a massage therapist who knows how to treat fibromyalgia during such times. In some patients, deep massage during a flare-up can exacerbate the pain. Therefore, deep tissue massage or any other form that works the deep muscles is not recommended during a flare-up.

MEDITATION

If your idea of meditation is sitting cross-legged on the floor in a room with burning incense, that could be one scenario, but it is not the norm. In fact, you can practice meditation just about anywhere: while taking a walk, washing the dishes, enjoying a sunset, or waiting for your kids at the bus stop. That's because there are many ways to meditate, which is wonderful because it has made meditation much more accessible to everyone, including people who have fibromyalgia.

Meditation can help fibromyalgia patients manage their

symptoms, improve their sleep, and lift their mood. Although there are many techniques, at its most basic level meditation consists of focusing on your breath or a certain sound, object, word, or activity in order to enter into an altered state of consciousness. During meditation you can achieve relaxation, release stress and tension from your mind and body, and quiet your mind. Other benefits include reduced heart rate, lowered blood pressure, fewer mood swings, increased memory, decreased levels of anxiety, and feeling more vitality.

In one study of 77 fibromyalgia patients, 51 percent of the participants reported moderate to marked improvement in their fibromyalgia symptoms. In another study, fibromyalgia patients who practiced meditation daily experienced fewer muscle aches and less sleeplessness, muscle pain, and depression. Sound appealing? Meditation requires no equipment, but you do need to be patient and to practice regularly for best results.

Walking Meditation for Fibromyalgia

One of the best forms of meditation for people with fibromyalgia is walking meditation. This form allows individuals to enjoy the benefits of both meditation and easy, low-impact exercise, which is so important for fibromyalgia patients.

In walking meditation, the act of walking is your focus. You become mindful of the experience of walking and try to keep your awareness focused on that experience. This differs from the traditional idea of meditation in several ways. An obvious one is that you keep your eyes open, and you also engage your world rather than withdraw your attention from it. You must be aware of your surroundings for reasons of safety, and because you are out moving in the environment, factors such as weather, sounds, and other people "invade" your meditation process.

Through all of this, however, in walking meditation your focus should remain on the process of walking. For example, you will mentally note each time you lift your lower legs and place your feet on the ground. Focus on the physical sensations that occur each time your feet touch the ground, the pressure on your heel, then your toes. Always keep your mind on the sensations of walking.

Do not watch your feet unless you must because there are obstacles on the ground. It is not helpful to focus on the image of your feet while you are trying to concentrate on the sensations in your legs and feet.

Walking meditation can be done any time you take a walk. If you prefer the more traditional form of meditation, there are many books, tapes, and Web sites that describe various ways to meditate. Regardless of the way you choose to meditate, numerous studies have shown that regular practice can help reduce stress, depression, and pain, and may help with sleep disturbances as well.

DID YOU KNOW?

Several studies have shown that mindfulness meditation can relieve some symptoms associated with fibromyalgia. Mindfulness meditation involves focusing your mind to be aware of your thoughts and actions in the present, without judging yourself. One study in Switzerland, for example, evaluated 52 women with fibromyalgia. The women were assigned to participate in eight weeks of mindfulness meditation practice or a social support procedure. Both immediately after the eight-week period and at a three-year follow-up, women who had participated in mindfulness meditation showed significantly better benefits regarding depression, anxiety, and the ability to cope with pain than did the women in the support group.

NEUROFEEDBACK

Have you heard of biofeedback? Like biofeedback, neuro-feedback is direct training of brain function that allows in-dividuals to consciously control their brain waves. It is also known as EEG biofeedback, because it is based on electrical brain activity, as is the electroencephalogram (EEG). It is simply biofeedback that is applied directly to the brain.

Here's how it works. A trained therapist—typically a psy-chologist, nurse, counselor, or rehab specialist—applies elec-trodes to your scalp. This allows the therapist to listen to your brain wave activity. Your brain wave activity is presented to you in the form of a video game, and you then essentially play a game with your brain, trying to alter your brain waves into a more favorable activity. When you change your brain waves correctly, you get a "reward," such as a certain sound.

The brain wave frequencies the therapist targets and the specific locations on the scalp where he or she listens to the waves are specific to the conditions you want to address. Es-sentially, the therapist can help you learn how to alter your brain waves, which in turn can cause the symptoms associ-ated with your old brain wave patterns—those associated with fibromyalgia symptoms—to disappear.

Although few studies have evaluated how effective neuro-feedback is in people who have fibromyalgia, it has been studied in individuals who suffer with chronic pain, depres-sion, anxiety, sleep disorders, chronic headache, and short-term memory loss—all symptoms seen in fibromyalgia. In a small study conducted in 2007, researchers used neurofeed-back in three patients with fibromyalgia. After 10 sessions, all the patients reported improvement in pain, fatigue, and depression. In a larger, earlier study conducted in Canada, people with fibromyalgia reported noticeable improvements in mental clarity, sleep, mood, and pain after participating in neurofeedback sessions.

Neurofeedback sessions typically last between 40 and 60

minutes, although your first session may be up to two hours. Your therapist and you can decide how many sessions per week will help you reach your goals. On average, most people experience improvements in their symptoms within the first 10 sessions.

If you find that neurofeedback really works for you, it is possible to get equipment you can use at home. Devices for home use can run off your home computer or a portable pack. A therapist can instruct you on how to use a home device and how to place the electrodes on your scalp, or there are helmets that have electrodes already attached. You can talk to your therapist about a home device.

MICHAEL'S EXPERIENCE WITH ALTERNATIVE THERAPIES

"I still can't believe I got this syndrome," says Michael, a 42-year-old engineer who spent three years looking for a diagnosis for his body pain, fatigue, fibrofog, depression, and headaches. "I really thought it just happened to women. I was really lucky to find a doctor who worked with me." Michael's three-year journey, however, led him to a place of uncertainty: how was he going to treat his symptoms so he could live his life to the fullest?

"I don't have anything against medications," he says, "but I don't want to have to depend on them, and I worry about side effects." Michael explained his concerns to his physician, who insisted that medications and exercise were the only "real" ways to treat his symptoms. "I didn't disagree with the exercise part, but I wasn't pleased with the verdict on the medications," Michael says. "I knew there had to be other options."

Michael did agree to take an antidepressant, which did provide some relief for his depression, and he chose to take over-the-counter pain relievers. While doing some research into other possible treatment strategies, he came across some

studies about acupuncture and chiropractic care in fibromyalgia patients. He was intrigued.

"Here were some options I was willing to try," he says. "I
found an acupuncture practitioner who used electroacupuncture, and after just a few sessions I felt improvement in
my level of pain." Michael continued to get acupuncture treatments every few weeks and also started a moderate walking
program, but also wanted to try chiropractic care which he
hoped would help his headaches. After several sessions with
a chiropractor, who performed some gentle adjustments,
Michael's headaches improved.

"I'm still not 100 percent," he says. "There are still some
days when it's hard to get out of bed because I'm so tired. But
I must say that the pain is much better, and I attribute that
to the acupuncture and chiropractic care. Oh, and I do walk
nearly every day. Next on my list of things to try is massage.
I'm hoping it will help me sleep and maybe I'll be able to
fight off this fatigue a little better."

THE BOTTOM LINE

Each of the alternative/complementary therapies discussed
in this chapter have provided significant relief for some
people who have fibromyalgia. One or more of them may do
the same for you. We hope you will review them, seek additional information from practitioners, organizations (see
"Resources"), and others who have tried these methods, and
find something that resonates with you.

CHAPTER EIGHT

Herbal Remedies and Nutritional Supplements

Managing the symptoms of fibromyalgia is a challenge, and so we like to bring in all the reinforcements we can. Among the possible treatment options are nutritional and herbal supplements. Many people with fibromyalgia report success when using these natural approaches to relieve different symptoms of fibromyalgia.

Few studies have explored the pros and cons of using natural supplements for various symptoms of fibromyalgia, but if there is anything positive about this syndrome, it is that it shares many symptoms with other conditions for which there are more studies of nutritional and herbal remedies. Therefore, in this chapter we include any scientific information on the use of natural supplements for fibromyalgia and, when that is lacking, evidence that various supplements can provide relief for symptoms associated with the syndrome.

In a University of Illinois at Chicago study published in May 2009 in the *Journal of Women's Health,* researchers questioned 434 women who reported having fibromyalgia and 198 women who did not. The researchers asked the women about their use of both medications and natural supplements. Forty-three percent of the women with fibromyalgia said they used at least one herb or nutritional supplement for their symptoms. The most popular supplements were omega-3 fatty acids, ginkgo, and glucosamine.

This chapter discusses what scientists know about these three supplements and numerous other herbal and nutritional therapies and their potential or actual impact on the syndrome. You will find many options in this chapter, and we suggest you read through them and then select two or three that match the symptoms you wish to address. We hope you will find one or more that you can use either alone or along with other treatment options to find relief from your symptoms.

WHY TRY NATURAL SUPPLEMENTS?

Some people with fibromyalgia, especially those who have not experienced much relief when using prescription medications or who cannot tolerate them, turn to nutritional and herbal supplements either to replace or to complement other therapies. One caveat about natural supplements to remember is that, like synthetic drugs, they can cause reactions in some people. They also can interact with any other medications you may be taking. That's why *we strongly recommend you inform your medical practitioner about any supplements you plan to take,* and that you also consult a holistic practitioner who uses alternative treatments to help you make the best choices for your needs.

Another word of caution is that pregnant women should not use herbal remedies, even though in the majority of cases there is no evidence that they are harmful. However, pregnant women should always check with their healthcare provider before they take any type of supplement or medication.

Having mentioned these cautionary notes, you should also know that natural treatments are typically associated with fewer and less severe side effects, and that they can be very helpful in relieving symptoms of fibromyalgia, especially when used along with mind/body approaches like those discussed in Chapter 7. A little patience is required, however, because the majority of nutrients and herbs take

some time, often several months, before you will notice benefits. Some take effect more quickly, like the calming effects
of chamomile.

Let's look at some of the more beneficial natural supplements for treating fibromyalgia symptoms.

ACES FOR ENERGY

A combination of four antioxidants—vitamins A, C, and E,
and the mineral selenium—is sometimes recommended to
help fight free-radical damage and inflammation, and to boost
energy levels. A suggested combination of doses includes
5,000 to 10,000 IU vitamin A, up to 10,000 buffered vitamin
C, 400 to 800 IU vitamin E, and 200 mcg selenium. Naturally, consult your physician before taking this combination
of antioxidants. If you are pregnant, plan to get pregnant, or
have liver disease, talk to your doctor before taking vitamin
A. Anyone who has high blood pressure should limit their
use of supplemental vitamin E to 400 IU daily, and anyone
who takes a blood thinner should not take vitamin E without
first talking to their healthcare provider.

B-COMPLEX

The B-complex family of vitamins includes eight essential
B vitamins: thiamine, riboflavin, niacin, pantothenic acid,
pyridoxine, folate, biotin, and cobalamin. Some supplements
also include a ninth vitamin, inositol. The majority of the B
family members are involved in energy production and metabolism, although they also play a role in the production of
hormones, red blood cells, and neurotransmitters. In some
cases several of the B vitamins must work in sync for a specific process to occur. If just one of the members is in short
supply, it can have a negative impact on energy production,

which can lead to fatigue and lethargy. Therefore, if you have fibromyalgia, the B vitamins are your friend.

Here's a snapshot of what each of the B vitamins can do for you.

- **Thiamine (B1).** This family member plays a role in the functioning of the nervous system and muscles, carbohydrate metabolism, enzyme processes, and the production of hydrochloric acid, which is necessary for proper digestion (and thus has a role in irritable bowel syndrome).

- **Riboflavin (B2).** The nervous system, energy production, and the formation of red blood cells are the tasks of this B vitamin. It has properties that can help reduce chronic fatigue and improve mood.

- **Niacin (B3).** Two different compounds are sometimes collectively given this name: nicotinic acid and niacinamide. Niacin is involved in energy production, while niacinamide can be used to treat arthritis.

- **Pantothenic acid (B5).** This is another energy production vitamin, and it also is involved in the manufacture of cholesterol, steroid hormones, hemoglobin, and melatonin.

- **Pyridoxine (B6).** This vitamin might be called the "Busy B," because it plays a role in more than 100 different enzyme systems. It also is involved in the synthesis of neurotransmitters in the brain, which is why it may help improve mood.

- **Biotin.** The synthesis and breakdown of amino acids, cholesterol, and fatty acids is the main task of this vitamin.

- **Folate.** Also known as folic acid to many people (folic acid is the synthetic form found in supplements; folate is the natural form found in foods), it works with vitamins B6 and B12 to control the level of homocysteine in the body. Homocysteine is a substance that plays a role in heart disease and stroke.

- **Cobalamin (B12).** This B vitamin helps keep red blood cells and nerve cells healthy, and it also assists in the production of DNA.

- **Inositol.** Cell membranes require inositol in order to stay healthy. Because cell membranes regulate the substances that go into and out of the cells, inositol plays a critically important function.

High-potency vitamin B-complex supplements differ in the amounts of each vitamin that they provide. Here are some typical ranges you will see in products on the market.

- Thiamin: 10 to 100 mg

- Riboflavin: 10 to 50 mg

- Niacin: 10 to 100 mg

- Pantothenic acid: 25 to 100 mg

- Vitamin B6: 25 to 100 mg

- Biotin: 100 to 300 mcg

- Folate: 400 mcg

- Vitamin BV-12: 400 mcg

• Inositol: There is no standard recommended dose for this B vitamin; however, 100 mg is typical. You should take an equal amount of choline when you take inositol and a B-complex supplement.

BLACK CURRANT SEED OIL

The black currant is a shrub that has an oil rich in essential fatty acids, including gamma linolenic acid (GLA; 17 percent) and alpha linolenic acid (ALA; 13 percent). Both of these fatty acids have been shown in studies to reduce inflammation in the joints, as well as promote and maintain the body's vital functions. These essential fatty acids are metabolized by the body into prostaglandins, substances that can block pain and assist in the proper functioning of the circulatory system.

Black currant seed oil is effective in treating chronic inflammatory condition, aches, and cramps. While there are no specific scientific studies of use of the oil in fibromyalgia patients, it has been studied in rheumatoid arthritis. Results show that the oil decreases morning stiffness in the joints.

You can buy black currant seed oil in capsules. A typical dose is one to three 500-mg capsules daily. Black currant seed oil is considered to be a very safe supplement, and except for rare allergic reactions, there are no major side effects associated with its use.

BOSWELLIA

Gum resin derived from the bark of the Boswellia tree is the source of this herbal remedy. Another name for this Ayurvedic herb is frankincense, and traditionally it has been used to treat arthritis, ulcerative colitis, coughs, and asthma. Boswellia gets its anti-inflammatory and painkiller effects from boswellic acid, the major component of the herb.

Although there are no scientific studies of boswellia used in fibromyalgia patients, it has been studied in people with osteoarthritis. In a study published in *Arthritis Research and Therapy,* researchers found that boswellia significantly reduced pain and improved physical function in people with osteoarthritis. The authors even suggested that boswellia may improve joint health by reducing the deterioration of cartilage.

Boswellia is available in tablets and capsules, and the usual dose is 300 to 400 mg three times daily. When shopping for boswellia supplements, look for products that contain 60 percent boswellic acid.

BROMELAIN

Bromelain is an enzyme that is found in pineapple stems. It was first introduced as a supplement in 1957, and it is best known for helping to relieve inflammation and pain associated with osteoarthritis.

In a head-to-head study of bromelain and the nonsteroidal anti-inflammatory drugs (NSAID) diclofenac in patients who had osteoarthritis of the hip, the two treatments provided similar pain and inflammation relief at the end of the six-week study. If you would like an effective alternative to NSAIDs, then bromelain may be your choice. A typical dose of the capsules or tablets is 500 to 2,000 mg three times daily between meals. Bromelain is also available in a cream that you can apply to painful areas of the body. Avoid bromelain, however, if you are allergic to pineapple. Bromelain can cause diarrhea and stomach upset.

CAPSAICIN

Cayenne (*Capsicum annuum*) has a long history of use among Native Americans, and it is an important spice in various cuisines throughout the world. It is also considered to be a medicine, and is a traditional herb in Ayurvedic, Chinese, Japanese, and Korean medicine as a treatment for digestive problems, circulatory problems, and arthritis and muscle pain.

The hot and spice nature of cayenne pepper is attributed mainly to a substance called capsaicin, which has pain-relieving abilities. Capsaicin's powers come from its ability to temporarily lower levels of substance P, an agent that promotes pain. When substance P levels are depleted, the pain signals no longer can reach the brain, and people feel relief. Specifically, it inhibits the neurotransmitters (chemicals in the brain) that are responsible for communicating pain signals.

Capsaicin is available in capsules and a cream, which can be applied topically to painful areas of the skin associated with fibromyalgia or arthritis. The cream should contain 0.025 to 0.075 percent capsaicin. For muscle pain, capsaicin cream can be applied several times a day. It typically takes three to seven days before you will notice any pain relief. In fact, when you first start using capsaicin your pain may increase slightly, but then it will diminish significantly over the next few days. If you are taking capsaicin capsules for digestive problems, the suggested dose is 30 to 120 mg taken three times daily.

CHAMOMILE

Why not sit down and enjoy a hot cup of chamomile tea? Chamomile (Roman chamomile) is one of the most calming herbs available. For people who have fibromyalgia, the relaxing effect of chamomile can promote sleep, which in turn may relieve other related fibromyalgia symptoms, such as pain, fatigue, and depression. Chamomile can also help relieve symptoms of anxiety, gastrointestinal upset (especially when related to stress), and menstrual cramps.

Chamomile is an herb you can pour from a teapot. Boil one teaspoon of Roman chamomile powder in eight ounces of water. Strain and drink the tea twice daily for one month, which is about how long it takes to enjoy most of the benefits of this herb, although a feeling of calm typically occurs much sooner. No side effects are associated with using Roman chamomile.

DEVIL'S CLAW

Devil's claw (*Harpagophytum procumbens*) is a South African herb with fruit that is covered with clawlike structures. It is the root, however, that holds the healing powers. Devil's claw has been used traditionally to treat arthritis, sore muscles, fever, and to help eliminate toxins from the blood. Studies show that devil's claw contains a chemical called harpagoside, which has anti-inflammatory powers. In one study of patients with osteoarthritis, devil's claw relieved pain as effectively as a commonly prescribed painkiller, while in another, the herb significantly reduced pain associated with rheumatic disorders and improved the patients' quality of life.

Devil's claw comes in tablets and liquid extract. Suggested doses are 0.2 to 0.25 mL of the liquid extract three times daily or 600 to 1,200 mg of tablets that have been standardized to contain 50 to 100 mg of harpagoside, also three times daily. Most people tolerate devil's claw well. Possible side effects include abnormal heart rhythms, headache, ringing in the ears, low blood pressure, and gastrointestinal upset. Because this herb theoretically may lower blood sugar levels, be cautious if you have diabetes.

GINGER

Ginger (*Zingiber officinale*) is a tropical plant whose underground stem (rhizome) is used as one of the most popular herbs in the world. For thousands of years, ginger has been used to treat nausea and stomachaches, diarrhea, arthritis, and heart conditions, and those uses still continue today.

Ginger contains several components which scientists believe are responsible for its healing qualities, including gingerols, shagaols, and some volatile oils. A study conducted at the University of Arizona in 2009 found that ginger provided a "very significant joint-protective effect" in animal models of rheumatoid arthritis. A subsequent study reported that 6-shagaol has a strong anti-inflammatory effect.

Ginger comes in several forms, including fresh, dried, or distilled oil from the rhizome. Suggested doses include 2 to 4 grams of fresh root daily or 30 to 90 drops of liquid extract daily. If you prefer tablets, use 75 to 2,000 mg of a product standardized to contain 4 percent volatile oils or 5 percent 6-gingerol or 6-shogaol. Teatime? Try steeping 2 tablespoons of freshly shredded ginger in boiling water for five to 10 minutes. Drink up to three cups daily.

Ginger usually does not cause side effects, but if you take more than the recommended amounts, you may experience mouth irritation, mild heartburn, and diarrhea. Do not take ginger if you have a bleeding disorder or if you are taking blood-thinning medication.

GINKGO

Ginkgo (*Ginkgo biloba*) is one of the most popular herbal remedies people turn to for fibromyalgia symptoms. The seeds of the ginkgo tree from which the herbal remedies are made have been used for about four thousand years as food and medicine to treat asthma, bronchitis, and brain disorders.

People with fibromyalgia use ginkgo because of its reported ability to enhance memory and brain function, and thus clear away fibrofog. As an antioxidant, ginkgo not only

DID YOU KNOW?

A study published in the April 26, 2010, online issue of the *Journal of Pain* reported on the effect of ginger on muscle pain. For 11 consecutive days, a total of 74 volunteers took either two grams of raw or heated ginger or a placebo. Then they performed various actions using their elbow flexors to induce pain and inflammation. The volunteers who had consumed either raw or heated ginger experienced about a 25 percent reduction in pain 24 hours after the exercise compared with the placebo group. Therefore, the authors concluded that daily supplementation with ginger can reduce muscle pain caused by exercise.

fights free-radical damage but also helps maintain the health of blood vessel walls, which improves blood flow to the brain and other parts of the body. Although there appears to be only one published scientific study on the ability of ginkgo to improve symptoms of fibromyalgia (and 64 percent of participants reported an improvement), others have looked at the benefits of ginkgo in improving overall brain function.

Thus far, research into the impact of ginkgo on cognition has provided mixed results, with some studies finding no benefit and others reporting an improvement in memory, mood, and depression. The findings of a 2009 meta-analysis of 36 studies that included ginkgo reported that "evidence that Ginkgo biloba has predicable and clinically significant benefit for people with dementia or cognitive impairment is inconsistent and unreliable."

Still, anecdotal reports from fibromyalgia patients are more positive. Whether there is a placebo effect happening or the herb is providing a benefit that experts have not been able to document for some reason remains to be seen. In the meantime, ginkgo is available as capsules, tablets, and tea. A typical dose is 80 to 240 mg of a standardized leaf extract taken daily in two to three divided doses. Look for supplements that have been standardized to 24 to 25 percent ginkgo flavone glycosides and 6 percent terpene lactones, the herb's active ingredients.

Possible side effects associated with ginkgo include diarrhea, dizziness, headache, gastrointestinal upset, and nausea. Because ginkgo may increase the risk of bleeding, do not use this herb if you are taking blood thinners or if you have a bleeding disorder.

GINSENG

When you hear the word "ginseng," it could refer to the American (*Anax quinquefolius*), the Korean or Asian (*Panax ginseng*), or the Siberian ginseng, which is not the same as the former two. Here we are talking about American and Asian ginseng, both of which contain ginsenosides, elements that provide the herb with its healing properties.

One of the strengths of ginseng is its ability to help the body cope with stress, a quality that makes it an adaptogen. Ginseng has been valued for millennia as an herb that boosts energy and relieves stress and tension, as well as acts as a "tonic" for the body—an immune system enhancer. Another traditional use is to stimulate and improve memory, which may help if you are suffering with fibrofog.

You can get ginseng in powders, tablets, liquid extracts, and capsules. Suggested doses are 100 to 200 mg, one to three times daily, of extract standardized to contain 4 to 5 percent ginsenosides. If you choose the liquid extract, you can take ¼ to ½ teaspoon one to three times daily. Ginseng should be taken with food.

Do not use ginseng for more than two to three weeks

continuously. Take a one-week break from ginseng before you resume taking it. Side effects are not common, but they may include insomnia, anxiety, diarrhea, vomiting, headache, nosebleed, and high blood pressure. If you are taking any medications to treat psychiatric disorders such as bipolar disorder or attention deficit hyperactivity disorder, ginseng may increase the effects of these medications, so consult your healthcare provider before starting the herb.

GLUCOSAMINE AND CHONDROITIN

Both glucosamine and chondroitin are popular natural treatment options for people who have fibromyalgia and arthritis, and for good reasons: they can reduce pain symptoms and also help increase joint strength.

Glucosamine is commonly used to help control joint pain and damage to cartilage in arthritis. Your body produces glucosamine naturally from glucose and an amino acid called glutamine. Its task in the body is to maintain cartilage and joint health. Glucosamine also works to create new cartilage cells.

Your body also produces chondroitin, another amino acid that is found inside the joint cartilage. Chondroitin helps to keep your joints lubricated by attracting and absorbing water, so they don't deteriorate. This substance also helps fight inflammation, which reduces pain.

Glucosamine and chondroitin often appear as a combination supplement, and both substances have been analyzed in many different studies, both separately and together. In fibromyalgia patients, the combination has helped relieve joint and muscle pain, reduce inflammation associated with related conditions such as rheumatoid arthritis and osteoarthritis, and increase joint strength and range of motion.

If you want to take glucosamine and chondroitin, either in combination or individually, consult your healthcare provider. Glucosamine supplements are typically made from shellfish (e.g., crab, lobster, shrimp), which should be avoided by anyone who has a shellfish allergy. Fortunately, several brands of glucosamine are now available from nonshellfish sources. Chondroitin supplements are made from either shark or cow cartilage.

A typical dose of glucosamine is 1,500 mg daily. If you weigh less than 100 pounds, your maximum dose should be 1,000 mg daily. Chondroitin is also taken daily at 900 to 1,200 mg, but the dose should be reduced if you weigh under 100 pounds. Regular use of glucosamine and chondroitin may cause intestinal gas, soft stools, nausea, and diarrhea.

5-HTP

5-hydroxytryptophan (5-HTP) is a derivative of the amino acid tryptophan and a building block of the powerful brain chemical serotonin. The body produces 5-HTP from the tryptophan found in certain foods, such as beef, chicken, fish, and other foods high in protein.

We have already talked about how serotonin plays a role in pain, mood, and sleep problems, and so maintaining a healthy level of this chemical is a critical part of relieving symptoms of fibromyalgia. Restoring serotonin levels to a healthy range is why people usually take antidepressants like selective serotonin reuptake inhibitors (SSRIs), and 5-HTP can produce a similar effect.

Supplements of 5-HTP work by increasing the synthesis of serotonin in the central nervous system. 5-hydroxytryptophan is the immediate precursor of serotonin, and the body readily absorbs oral supplements. Several studies have shown that people who take 5-HTP experience significant improvement in their symptoms.

Studies of the use of 5-HTP that specifically focus on people who have fibromyalgia are scarce, although one published in the *Alternative Medicine Review* found that the supplements improved symptoms of insomnia, pain, depression, and anxiety in fibromyalgia patients. Other studies have revealed 5-HTP to be effective in relieving symptoms typically experienced by people with fibromyalgia—even though the study subjects were not suffering from that condition.

A 2010 placebo-controlled study, for example, reported that use of a supplement that contained both 5-HTP and another amino acid, GABA, was very helpful for people who were experiencing sleep problems. The combination reduced time to fall asleep, improve quality of sleep, and increased how long people were able to stay asleep. Research from several sources show that 5-HTP is effective in relieving symptoms of depression.

Not every study of 5-HTP and the symptoms associated with fibromyalgia have produced positive results. However, many people have and still enjoy relief when using this supplement. Possible side effects of 5-HTP use include gastrointestinal disturbances such as heartburn, nausea, gas, diarrhea, constipation, and a rumbling stomach. Some people experience mild headache, rash, flushing, or vivid dreams. In rare cases it can cause high blood pressure, ulcers, irritable bowel syndrome, liver and lung disease, and blood disorders such as anemia and hemophilia.

DID YOU KNOW?

A study released in June 2010 found that serotonin levels in people with fibromyalgia were about 45 percent lower than those in healthy individuals. An important correlation was seen between serotonin levels and the severity of pain, depression, and the impact of the disease on quality of life, as well as on age.

If you are already taking any type of medication or other supplements, consult your healthcare provider before you begin taking 5-HTP. You should not take 5-HTP if you are also using any of the following: antidepressants, antibiotics, weight loss medications, tranquilizers, barbiturates, cancer chemotherapy drugs, anti-Parkinson's medications, or alcoholic beverages.

MAGNESIUM AND MALIC ACID

The mineral magnesium, along with malic acid, can help boost your energy and relieve fibromyalgia pain. Magnesium has a reputation for treating migraine, insomnia, and depression, as well as symptoms of premenstrual syndrome and chronic fatigue syndrome. Malic acid, which is a fruit acid extracted from apples, is critical in the formation of ATP, the body's energy source. Malic acid helps the body make ATP more efficiently. When you bring these two important substances together, it creates a winning combination.

The magnesium and malic acid combination works because these nutrients are precursors to the Krebs cycle, a series of reactions that occur in your body that are critical for the production of energy. Some people with fibromyalgia find that when they take 100 to 200 mg of magnesium and 400 to 800 mg of malic acid three times daily, about 20 minutes before each meal, they are better able to do their exercises and have energy left for the rest of the day. Generally, you should notice an improvement in pain within 48 hours of starting magnesium/malic acid, while it will likely take two weeks or more for fatigue to improve.

You can boost your magnesium intake by eating foods that are high in this mineral. These include nuts, sunflower seeds, barley, quinoa, bananas, pineapple, artichokes, avocados, lima beans, spinach, okra, hummus, cod, and sole.

Check with a knowledgeable healthcare provider to find the best combination for you. People who have heart or kidney problems should not take magnesium until they check with their doctor.

MELATONIN

To tackle sleep problems, you might try melatonin. This hormone is produced naturally by the body by the pineal gland in the brain, and it is also available as an over-the-counter supplement. Scores of studies show that it can induce drowsiness and improve sleep patterns for people who suffer with insomnia.

Melatonin can tackle sleep problems because one of its main tasks is to maintain the body's circadian rhythm, the 24-hour internal clock that helps regulate your wake/sleep cycle. Since lack of sleep and fatigue go hand in hand, especially in fibromyalgia patients, taking melatonin may offer some relief from both symptoms. Melatonin also plays a part in the timing and release of female reproductive hormones, so if you are experiencing menstruation problems, melatonin may help with these as well.

Because low doses appear to be just as effective as higher ones, the suggested starting dose is 0.3 mg per day, which is about what the body makes naturally. You and your healthcare provider can decide on raising the dose gradually if needed. Melatonin is available in both quick-release and sustained-release forms, and the jury is still out on which one produces better results.

Possible side effects include vivid dreams, dizziness, headache, irritability, stomach cramps, and reduced libido. It may also worsen symptoms of depression.

MSM

Methylsulfonylmethane (MSM) is a supplemental form of sulfur, a mineral that is found in eggs, fish, and many plants. Studies show that some people who have fibromyalgia have low or deficient levels of sulfur. Taking MSM can help correct that deficiency. Overall, however, MSM is important for keeping your connective tissues and joints healthy, and there is evidence that it can slow nerve signals that carry pain messages, which can reduce pain.

Some of the benefits you may experience from taking MSM include reduced muscle soreness and pain, enhanced blood circulation, improved digestion, and better immune system functioning. When MSM is taken along with glucosamine and chondroitin, the combination can better transport nutrients to damaged tissue and cartilage.

MSM is available as tablets, capsules, powders, crystals, and topical creams or gels. A common starting dose is 500 mg daily, which can be increased gradually to 1,000 mg and more, depending on your symptoms. MSM is very well tolerated even at high doses of 10 grams, but most people say they get relief between four and eight grams daily, which equals one to two teaspoons if you are taking the dried form. MSM works best if you drink lots of water throughout the day.

NADH

Nicotinamide adenine dinucleotide hydrogen (NADH) is an antioxidant enzyme that can be found in all living cells. One of its critical tasks is to facilitate the production of neurotransmitters such as dopamine and noradrenaline, which are often found in low levels in people who have fibromyalgia. Some fibromyalgia patients experience an improvement in energy level, concentration, and stamina when taking NADH supplements.

No studies have specifically evaluated NADH in fibromyalgia patients, but several have explored its effectiveness in individuals who have chronic fatigue syndrome. The results were positive, with 31 percent of patients in one study achieving significant improvement in energy and fatigue over time compared with only eight percent of patients on a placebo.

A typical dose of NADH is 15 mg taken 30 minutes before breakfast and dinner, but you should talk to your healthcare provider before taking this supplement. Some studies have used only 10 mg and had positive results.

OMEGA-3 FATTY ACIDS

Omega-3 essential fatty acids belong to a larger class of fats called polyunsaturated fats. The three omega-3s you hear the most about are eicosapentaenoic acid (EPA), docosahexaenoic acid (DHA), and alpha-linolenic acid (ALA). Every cell in your body needs omega-3s because these fatty acids keep cell membranes flexible, which permits nutrients to easily enter your cells.

Perhaps the most important benefit of omega-3s for people with fibromyalgia is the ability of these fatty acids to reduce inflammation, and in the process, reduce pain. The fatty acid also can help relieve depression. Studies show that most people do not get enough omega-3s from their food, as they are found mainly in certain cold-water fish such as tuna, salmon, and sardines. Other sources include flaxseed, walnuts, and pumpkin seeds. To boost omega-3 intake and also help fight inflammation, some people turn to fish oil supplements.

If the thought of taking fish oil does not appeal to you, an option is flaxseed oil supplements, which provide ALA. Although the body can more readily use EPA and DHA from both fish and supplements, it can use ALA to make EPA and DHA. Because the conversion rate of ALA to EPA and DHA is only 5 to 25 percent, you would need to take five to six times more ALA than taking fish oil alone. Don't worry: one tablespoon of flaxseed oil is packed with 8,000 mg of ALA, an excellent amount to take for fibromyalgia.

If you are considering taking fish oil, the amount you take depends on how much EPA and DHA are in the supplement. A common amount in fish oil capsules is 180 mg (0.18 grams) of EPA and 120 mg (0.12 grams) of DHA. If you see a 1,000 mg fish oil capsule, you need to check how much EPA and DHA it contains. A suggested daily amount of EPA and DHA combined is 300 to 500 mg, plus an additional 800 to 1,100 mg of ALA.

When you shop for fish oil supplements, look for brands that are labeled free of toxins or mercury-free, although this is not a guarantee that the product is toxic-free. Possible side effects of fish oil supplements include flatulence, belching, diarrhea, and a slightly fishy body odor. You can reduce or eliminate all these symptoms if you take the supplement with meals. It is also recommended that you start at a lower dose than recommended and increase it gradually.

PROBIOTICS

If you are experiencing digestive or intestinal symptoms, probiotics may help you. Probiotics are dietary supplements that contain beneficial bacteria. These microorganisms have the ability to assist with the breakdown of food, absorption of nutrients, and improve gastrointestinal challenges such as irritable bowel syndrome, a common problem in fibromyalgia. Probiotics also have been shown to effectively treat diarrhea, prevent and treat urinary tract infections, and help boost the immune system.

Probiotics work by helping to restore a healthy balance of "good" versus "bad" bacteria in the intestinal tract. Both beneficial and disease-causing bacteria can coexist in the intestinal tract, but for good overall health, you want a balance in favor of the good kind. The two main types of beneficial bacteria are *Lactobacillus* and *Bifidobacterium,* with numerous species in each genus that have been identified as being helpful.

Probiotics are dosed in units called CFUs—colony-forming units—and a typical dose can be one to two billion to 50 billion CFUs per day, depending on whether you are treating a condition or maintaining overall health. To fight active digestive symptoms, 50 billion CFUs several times a day may be needed at first. Once your symptoms improve, you can gradually decrease the dose. Many experts recommend taking a probiotic supplement that contains two or more species of beneficial bacteria.

Possible side effects associated with taking probiotics include mild gas or bloating, which usually subside after your body gets used to having a balanced intestinal tract!

S-ADENOSYLMETHIONINE (SAM-E)

SAM-e is a synthetic form of a compound that the body makes naturally from the amino acid methionine and adenosine triphosphate (ATP), an energy-producing molecule. Every cell in your body contains SAM-e, and it has a role in more than 100 different processes to maintain your health. Because the body produces less and less SAM-e as you age, some people take SAM-e supplements to treat symptoms that typically appear with advancing age.

Studies show that SAM-e can reduce the number of trigger points, reduce fatigue, and improve symptoms of depression. One of SAM-e's properties is the ability to protect the joints and promote the formation of cartilage. SAM-e also can reduce pain and inflammation, which can improve your range of motion and mobility. Experts believe SAM-e has these qualities because it increases the availability of two neurotransmitters that are involved in mood and pain, serotonin and dopamine. Studies that have compared SAM-e with antidepressants, such as imipramine, have shown that SAM-e provided comparable results and had few or no side effects.

SAM-e is available as tablets and capsules. The suggested dose is 400 mg two or three times daily, but ask your healthcare provider for the dose that best suits your needs. The optimal time to take SAM-e is two hours before or three hours after a meal, as the body absorbs it best on an empty stomach. Some people experience some heartburn or nausea, but this can be avoided if you take SAM-e with lots of water. Rarely, SAM-e may cause dry mouth, thirst, increased urination, headache, anxiety, and blood in the stool.

SAM-e can begin to provide benefits in as little as one to two weeks, while antidepressants traditionally take at least two weeks, and often four to six weeks before there are any significant results. Do not take SAM-e near the end of the day because it can cause a mild boost in energy and make it difficult to sleep. SAM-e can be used along with other natural antidepressants such as St. John's wort, as well as prescription antidepressants, but only under strict medical supervision. Take a high-potency vitamin B-complex supplement when taking SAM-e, because when SAM-e breaks down in the body, it forms an amino acid called homocysteine, which can cause heart problems if the levels reach high concentrations.

ST. JOHN'S WORT

St. John's wort (*Hypericum perforatum*) is a plant with yellow flowers whose medicinal powers were first noted by the ancient Greeks. Today the flowers are used to prepare teas and other forms of the supplement. St. John's wort is one of the most popular herbal remedies in the United States. Perhaps best known for its ability to help relieve symptoms of depression, St. John's wort can also help restore healthy sleep patterns.

St. John's wort can regulate levels of the neurotransmitters serotonin, dopamine, and norepinephrine, which have an impact on mood and pain. The two active ingredients believed to be responsible for these benefits are hypericin and pseudohypericin.

Although there are no studies that specifically evaluate the effect of St. John's wort in fibromyalgia patients, others have found the herb to be useful in treating depression, a common symptom of the syndrome. In fact, it's been shown to be as effective as tricyclic antidepressants in short-term treatment of mild or moderate depression, and as effective as selective serotonin reuptake inhibitors (SSRIs) such as Prozac in treating depression.

St. John's wort is available in capsules, tablets, tinctures, and teas. Choose supplements that are standardized to contain 0.3 percent hypericin. The typical dose of capsules and tablets is 300 to 500 mg three times daily. Liquid extracts can be taken at a dose of 40 to 60 drops twice daily. St. John's wort should be taken with meals. To prepare the tea, add one to two teaspoons of dried herb to eight ounces of boiling water. Allow the herb to steep for 10 minutes. Drink up to two cups daily. It can take up to eight weeks before you experience benefits from St. John's wort.

Most people tolerate St. John's wort well. The more common side effects are stomach upset, dry mouth, dizziness, headache, fatigue, and skin reactions. It may also cause your skin to become overly sensitive to sunlight. Do not take St. John's wort while taking antidepressants, as the combination may cause nausea, anxiety, headache, and confusion.

TURMERIC

Turmeric (*Curcuma longa*) is a plant native to South Asia and a member of the ginger family. It has been used for 4,000 years to treat various health conditions, mostly involving the gastrointestinal tract. The active substance in turmeric is called curcumin, and it is said that it stimulates the gallbladder to produce bile, which in turn can improve digestion. In fact, at least one double-blind, placebo-controlled study showed that turmeric reduced gas and bloating in people who had indigestion, and another showed that it was effective in treating irritable bowel syndrome.

Turmeric also reduces inflammation, which in turn can relieve pain, including pain that accompanies fibromyalgia and arthritis. Studies suggest that turmeric may be as effective as cortisone in relieving pain, but without the drug's side effects.

Turmeric is available in capsules, fluid extract, and tincture. If you choose capsules with standardized powder (curcumin), a typical dose is 400 to 600 mg, three times daily. The fluid extract dose is usually 30 to 90 drops daily. Turmeric and curcumin are safe when taken at the recommended doses. Large amounts of turmeric for long periods of time may cause an upset stomach. If you have diabetes, you should talk to your doctor before using turmeric, because it may lower your blood sugar levels.

VALERIAN

If you are looking for help with sleep disturbances, valerian may be the herb for you. This native plant of Europe and Asia contains the active ingredients valerenic acid and bornyl, which are derived from the essential oil in its roots. Most supplements contain standardized valerenic acid. This substance is believed to be responsible for valerian's impact on a neurotransmitter called GABA in the central nervous system, and for the herb's tranquilizing effect.

Valerian is most commonly used to help people sleep and to treat anxiety. Results of studies of individuals who experience sleep disturbances have been mixed. One well-designed study found that valerian was no more effective than a placebo in improving sleep for the first 28 days of the study, but after that valerian significantly improved sleep. Thus the researchers concluded that people may need to take the herb for several weeks before it begins to be effective. Some studies indicate that valerian reduces the time it takes to fall asleep and improves sleep quality.

A typical dose is 150 to 300 mg extract standardized to contain 0.8 percent valerenic acid, or ¼ to ½ teaspoon valerian tincture several times daily. When valerian is used at the recommended dose, the risk of side effects is very low. Some people experience stomachache, and at large doses it can cause headache, nausea, grogginess in the morning, and restlessness. You should not take valerian for longer than two months because at that point it can cause insomnia. If you have been taking high doses of valerian for several months, you could experience withdrawal symptoms (e.g., confusion, rapid heartbeat) if you stop taking it abruptly.

VITAMIN D

Vitamin D, the sunshine vitamin, has a direct association with chronic pain. This is a very significant finding, because it means that correcting deficiencies of this vitamin—and most people have low or deficient levels of vitamin D—can provide some positive feedback for people with fibromyalgia.

Research conducted under the auspices of the Mayo Clinic has revealed that people with chronic pain who take narcotic medications such as oxycodone, morphine, or fentanyl at high amounts have the greatest deficiencies of vitamin D, while those taking lower doses of narcotics had adequate levels of the vitamin. This indicated to scientists that there is something about vitamin D that reduces the need for pain medication—and thus it must somehow reduce pain.

Although many people know that vitamin D has an important role in bone health and in developing muscle strength, few have realized that a deficiency of vitamin D is associated with widespread pain and poor neuromuscular function. Michael Turner, MD, of the Mayo Comprehensive Pain Rehabilitation Center in Rochester, Minnesota, studies patients with chronic pain and assessed their vitamin D levels. Turner's findings, which were published in *Pain Medicine* in 2008, led him to say that "many patients who have been labeled with fibromyalgia are, in fact, suffering from symptomatic vitamin D inadequacy."

This finding has been supported by subsequent studies. In one from the University of Manchester in May 2010, the investigators found that men with chronic widespread musculoskeletal pain had a 50 percent increased chance of having inadequate levels of vitamin D than men who did not have chronic pain.

This is all good news, if only because vitamin D deficiency is easy to correct. One of the tests your healthcare provider performs should be a blood test to determine your vitamin D level. Once that has been determined, you can decide how to correct any deficiency. One way is to get exposure to direct sunlight (without wearing sunscreen) for 10 to 15 minutes at least four days per week. One drawback is that not all sunlight is created equal, so to speak: the closer you are to the equator, the better the quality of the sunlight. If you live in more northern latitudes, such as in Chicago or Portland, Oregon, then the sun quality is not as good in terms of vitamin D production.

Even if you do get some sun exposure, a vitamin D supplement may be in order. Your healthcare provider can determine what dose you need, depending on the severity of your deficiency. Some people find that once they correct any vitamin D deficiency, 1,000 IU daily is a healthy maintenance dose. But how much vitamin D do you need?

According to the Vitamin D Council and other experts,

the ideal blood level of vitamin D is between 50 and 80 ng/mL (nanograms per milliliter). Among conventional American medical circles, 30 ng/mL is considered "normal." The majority of Americans are deficient by Vitamin D Council standards, because their levels are around 30 ng/mL or lower. To increase their blood levels of vitamin D, the Council recommends that people take 5,000 IU daily for 2 to 3 months, then ask their doctor for a vitamin D test to identify their levels. Why are levels between 50 and 80 ng/mL so important? Research shows that the body cannot begin to adequately store vitamin D until the nutrient reaches a level of at least 50 ng/mL. Below that, the body uses up the vitamin as fast as it makes it or takes it in.

LYNDA'S NATURAL FIGHT AGAINST FIBROMYALGIA

At age 51, Lynda has long had a reputation as a fighter. As an attorney, she has donated thousands of hours to represent people who could not afford a lawyer but who were fighting for causes Lynda believes are just, such as animal and environmental rights. So when she was sidelined in her late 40s with overwhelming fatigue, pain, insomnia, and problems with concentration, she was furious. "I didn't have time to not feel well," she says. "Too many people were depending on me, and I wanted to represent my clients and their causes to the best of my ability. Except I felt my abilities slipping away."

Lynda was fortunate in that she found a rheumatologist within just a few months who diagnosed her with fibromyalgia, but his "verdict" that she needed to take medications to fight her battle did not sit right with her. At first she "gave in" and took pregabalin (Lyrica), but the side effects were too intolerable. Encouraged by studies that said exercise was helpful, she went to a physical therapist and established a daily exercise program she was able to do at home and at a gym. But while the exercise helped, it was not enough. Lynda was still "off my game," and she decided to investigate more.

Her searching led her to try a combination of natural supplements which, with the help of a naturopath, she narrowed down to four: vitamin D, omega-3 fatty acids, glucosamine/chondroitin, and MSM. After about a month of adjusting the dosages of these four supplements, she began feeling better. "My pain improved significantly," she says, "and as the pain decreased I was better able to exercise, which seemed to improve my fatigue." Next she added 5-HTP to help with her insomnia, and then she felt she had found the right combination of nutrients to help her with her fight.

"I have more good days than bad, and I'm really happy that I'm able to handle the fibromyalgia without taking prescription drugs. Although I do take acetaminophen occasionally, that's about all in the way of drugs. When I need a real pick-me-up, I get a massage. Most days I can fight for my clients while still fighting the fibromyalgia, and that makes me feel great."

THE BOTTOM LINE

Nutritional supplements and herbal remedies can be effective complementary treatments for a variety of fibromyalgia symptoms. Consult a knowledgeable healthcare practitioner before starting any new nutritional or herbal supplement, and record your experiences with him or her in your journal. Because the positive effects of natural supplements typically take longer to experience than those associated with medications, it is good to have a written record of your start times and your progress to help you and your doctor determine the effects of these supplements.

CHAPTER NINE

Fighting Fibromyalgia With Diet

In the fight against fibromyalgia, one way you can make an impact on your symptoms and overall well-being every day, several times a day, is with your food choices. Although there is no "official" diet for fighting fibromyalgia, there are some thoughtful guidelines as well as lots of anecdotal evidence that selected approaches have shown some benefits.

One reason there is no one fibromyalgia diet is that the syndrome involves so many symptoms and conditions that differ from person to person. Many fibromyalgia patients, for example, have irritable bowel syndrome, which generally means those individuals should avoid simple sugars (including those in fruits) and milk products while enjoying high-fiber foods, including whole grains, to improve symptoms of constipation and diarrhea. Yet fibromyalgia patients without irritable bowel syndrome often can enjoy healthy fruits without any problems, while those who have celiac disease need to avoid most grain products. So establishing "the" fibromyalgia diet is not possible.

However, that does not mean you can't experience relief from your symptoms if you decide to follow a certain dietary path that has proven helpful to some people. You may also discover that the best diet for you is one that suggests you eliminate a specific list of foods which some experts have found to have a negative impact on people who have fibromyalgia. Indeed, many fibromyalgia patients have enjoyed symptom relief by making changes in their diet, changes that have not only improved their pain and energy levels, but also their overall health and quality of life.

In this chapter we explore some dietary basics that have been researched by experts and found to be helpful for people who have fibromyalgia, as well as several specific dietary plans that have proved beneficial for some patients. The important thing to remember is that each person who has fibromyalgia is unique, and so the dietary choices you make will be ones that suit *your* specific needs and symptoms.

A GENERAL DIETARY APPROACH FOR FIBROMYALGIA

Generally, a good dietary foundation for people who have fibromyalgia is an eating plan that focuses on lots of fresh fruits and vegetables and whole-grain foods, is low in saturated fat, includes fish rich in omega-3 fatty acids, and limits the amount of meat and poultry (lean only) and low-fat dairy. Although this general approach will not necessarily reduce your fibromyalgia symptoms, it can help to reduce the risk of other conditions that can make your syndrome worse.

Another reason to focus on a nutrient-rich diet is to feed your mitochondria. The mitochondria are the energy-producing portions of your cells, and, as we mentioned in Chapter 2, mitochondrial dysfunction is a possible cause of the fatigue that affects people with fibromyalgia. Therefore it is important to maintain a high level of nutrients to keep your mitochondria properly "fueled."

FOODS THAT WORK FOR YOU

When we talked about causes of pain in fibromyalgia in Chapter 2, one factor we mentioned was how oversensitive nerve cells in the brain and spinal cord affect the way fibromyalgia patients process pain. Certain foods and components of foods or additives may trigger the release of neurotransmitters that can enhance a person's sensitivity to pain. Therefore, one strategy you can try is to focus on foods that do not trigger this pain process. Here are some eating strategies that will not only provide you with important nutrients, but also may improve your quality of life.

- **Fresh foods.** Foods that have no preservatives or artificial additives are not only healthy overall, they also may relieve symptoms of fibromyalgia that are associated with irritable bowel syndrome, which affects more than half of fibromyalgia patients. Fresh, natural foods also are "cleaner," which means you expose your body to less pain-promoting toxins. Focus on a whole foods diet, one as free of processed, refined, and fast food as possible, and your body will definitely benefit from those efforts.

- **Foods rich in omega-3 fatty acids.** The best sources of these foods are certain fatty fish like salmon, tuna, and herring, as well as flaxseed, walnuts, and some fortified cereals. What's the secret behind omega-3s? They fight inflammation, and inflammation often causes pain. Although there have not been any studies that specifically explored the impact of omega-3s in fibromyalgia patients, the fatty acids are effective in relieving pain and inflammation in a closely related condition, arthritis.

- **Eat every few hours.** Small meals with one or two intermittent small snacks can help you maintain your energy level (and not let your blood sugar levels drop too low), and also keep your metabolism at its maximum. If you let yourself get too hungry, it is too easy to overeat at your next meal, and may cause you to eat unhealthy foods.

- **Choose nutritious snacks.** Fresh raw fruits and vegetables, whole-grain crackers, dried fruit, vegetable juices, dry roasted unsalted nuts (in small amounts), a green tea smoothie (see "Did You Know?" on page 170), no- or low-fat plain yogurt with fresh fruit, and popcorn without butter are good choices.

- **Love those complex carbs!** Complex carbohydrates should make up about 55 to 60 percent of your daily caloric intake. One reason complex carbs are so important is that they provide most of the fuel your body needs for energy and to help heal your muscles. Replace the simple carbohydrates in your diet with complex ones, and you should notice an increase in energy (and possibly a drop in weight as well).

- **Choose power protein.** This macronutrient should make up 15 percent of your calories. Vegetable proteins are more healthful than animal-based proteins for people who have fibromyalgia, as they are lower in saturated fat, have no cholesterol, and contain fiber. In addition, conventionally raised meats contain antibiotics, hormones, and other additives that are best avoided by everyone, and especially people who have fibromyalgia.

- **Be choosy about fats.** Fat should make up 25 to 30 percent of your calories. Although fats often get a bad name, the healthful ones—monounsaturated fats, omega-3 fatty acids, and some polyunsaturated fats—are a wise and essential addition to your diet. Make sure the majority of your fats come from this group, while minimizing saturated fats and avoiding trans fats.

- **Make friends with fiber.** Most American adults eat only about half of the recommended 25 to 35 grams of fiber per day. Getting enough fiber is especially important for people who have fibromyalgia, as up to 75 percent of them have irritable bowel syndrome, and fiber can ease the symptoms. Fiber is the part of plants that the body cannot digest, which is great because it helps transport foods and toxins through the digestive tract and out of the body. There are two types of fiber: insoluble, which helps promote regular bowel movements and eliminates toxins; and soluble, which helps lower cholesterol and protect the heart. About one-quarter of your daily fiber intake should come from soluble fiber and the rest from insoluble fiber. Fiber-rich foods typically contain both types, although one type dominates (see chart below).

- **Drink purified water.** Sometimes it is hard to remember to drink water, but if you keep several reusable water bottles in the refrigerator, you will always have one ready to take with you whenever you leave the house. Also keep a pitcher of purified water in your refrigerator, with lemon if you prefer.

- **Eat slowly.** Take time to thoroughly chew and enjoy your food. Digestion does not begin in your stomach: it begins in your mouth. Since chewing is the initial step, if you do not chew your food well, it begins its journey through the rest of your digestive tract on the wrong foot, contributing to indigestion, gas, bloating, and pain. And more pain is not what you need!

- **Prepare foods in healthful ways.** Steam vegetables lightly to help retain their nutrients. Broiled and baked fish and poultry are the most healthful ways to cook them. Avoid frying foods, and do not grill meat until it is charred or burnt, because it can transform the amino acids in the meat into carcinogens.

FIBER-RICH FOODS
AND HOW TO EAT MORE OF THEM

Although the suggested intake of fiber is 25 percent soluble and 75 percent insoluble, the most important thing is simply to get enough fiber, period.

Soluble Fiber: Apples, berries, broccoli, cabbage, carrots, cauliflower, citrus, dates, dried beans, flaxseed, lentils, oats/oat bran, peas, pumpkin, squash, sweet potatoes

Insoluble fiber: Fruit skins, most vegetables, nuts, root vegetable skins, seeds, whole-grain products

You can get more fiber in your diet if you:

• eat raw vegetables for snacks.

• choose breakfast cereals that contain more than three grams of fiber per serving.

• eat beans or legumes every day. Try adding them to soups, salads, and casseroles.

• add dried fruit to your oatmeal or dry cereal.

• keep the skins on your fruits and vegetables (buy organic when possible and always thoroughly wash any produce, organic or conventional, before eating).

• always choose whole-grain breads, pasta, crackers, and other grain products.

DID YOU KNOW?

Some foods can help boost your levels of scrotonin, the brain chemicals that can help improve mood and reduce pain. Examples include (all whole-grain) bagels, breads, cereals, crackers, muffins, and pasta. Others include brown rice and potatoes (but not fried!).

FABULOUS FOODS FOR FIBROMYALGIA

This is a suggested list of foods. As we have already noted, some people with fibromyalgia have no problems with, say, whole grains, while others do. It is up to you to experiment and find the most nutritious, fabulous foods that work best for your body.

Power Proteins

Amaranth (a complete protein grain)
Beans (e.g., black, pinto, white, garbanzo, navy)
Cheese (low-fat, organic)
Chicken and turkey breast (organically raised)
Egg whites
Herring
Lentils
Nuts (in small portions)
Quinoa (a complete protein grain)
Salmon
Sardines
Seeds (in small portions)
Soybeans and soy-based foods
Split peas
Tuna

Complex Carbohydrates

Apples
Banana
Barley
Berries (blueberries, raspberries, strawberries)
Bread (whole-grain)
Brown rice
Couscous
Corn
Mango
Millet
Oatmeal
Papaya
Pasta (whole-grain)
Sweet potatoes
Squash
Wild rice
Yams

Vegetables

Asparagus
Bell peppers (green, red, orange, yellow)
Broccoli
Brussels sprouts
Cabbage
Carrots
Cauliflower
Cucumbers
Green beans
Greens (kale, mustard greens, turnip greens, Romaine lettuce, spinach)
Onions
Peas
Tomatoes

DID YOU KNOW?

You can get the nutrition benefits of green tea (it is high in antioxidants) in a great-tasting smoothie, and it's low in calories, too. Brew one cup of green tea and chill it (or brew ½ cup and add ½ cup ice cubes to chill it). Place the green tea in a blender or food processor along with ½ banana and one peeled, pitted, sliced peach. Blend until smooth. If you like a little sweetness, add a pinch of stevia.

Healthy Fats

Evening primrose oil
Flaxseeds and oil
Olive oil
Pumpkin seeds and oil
Sesame oil
Sunflower seeds and oil

FOODS AND ADDITIVES TO AVOID

Along with focusing on an overall healthy diet, there are certain foods and food additives that appear to have a negative impact on a significant number of people with fibromyalgia. Approximately 70 to 80 percent of the foods most Americans eat are processed in some way, which means synthetic ingredients such as artificial colors, flavors, preservatives, and other chemicals have been added.

Since the Food and Drug Administration (FDA) allows more than 10,000 food and chemical additives to be put into the food supply, it is not possible to address them all here. Many of these added ingredients have not been studied adequately to be sure they are completely safe for human consumption, yet they are allowed to be added to food products. Generally, it is best to avoid food additives as much as possible, which means focusing on fresh, organically grown foods and other foods that have been minimally processed.

We have compiled a short list of foods and additives that can exacerbate symptoms in people who have fibromyalgia. Avoiding these items does not guarantee your symptoms will go away or even change, but it is certainly worth eliminating at least a few of these foods or additives to see what happens. You could be very pleasantly surprised!

Aspartame

You may know it better as NutraSweet, but it isn't so sweet on fibromyalgia patients. At least one study, published in the *Annals of Pharmacotherapy* in 2001, showed that eliminating aspartame from the diet of fibromyalgia patients resulted in an improvement of symptoms. Aspartame is classified as an excitotoxin, which is known to stimulate pain receptors. When pain changes from acute to chronic, a pain receptor called NMDA opens up. Aspartame helps to stimulate this opening. Another study reported that people with fibromyalgia have an abundance of NMDA receptors in their skin, which increases the possibility of pain. Eliminating aspartame is worth a try, and if you really need another noncaloric sugar substitute, try the natural herb stevia.

BHA and BHT

Butylated hydroxyanisole (BHA) and butylated hydroxytoluene (BHT) are preservatives that are often added to a wide variety of foods. BHA is found mainly in products such as baked goods, candy, soup bases, breakfast cereals, shortening, dry mixes for desserts, potato flakes, and ice cream. BHT inhibits rancidity in frozen and fresh pork sausage and freeze-dried meats, and it is also used in shortenings and chewing gum. Both BHA and BHT can form potentially cancer-causing reactive compounds in the body. Other side effects of these food additives include immune disorders, liver and kidney damage, infertility, and elevated cholesterol.

Caffeine

Doesn't a steaming cup of rich coffee sound like just the right thing to perk you up? How about a can of cola? Yes, these caffeine-laden beverages can give you a quick pick-me-up, but like sugary foods, the high is quick and the fall is hard. In fact, with caffeine the "down" is a sedative effect. When you have fibromyalgia you are already tired, and the sedative effect of the caffeine only makes the fatigue more intense and longer lasting. The promising news is that once people cut out caffeine, they often experience an improvement in their fatigue within a week.

Dairy Products

Dairy foods, especially milk, have been known to exacerbate symptoms of fibromyalgia. If you are lactose intolerant, dairy products can worsen your fibromyalgia symptoms. Dairy is also one of the more common food allergies, and if you are allergic to milk products, eating them will only worsen your symptoms. There are also many anecdotal reports that eliminating dairy products can relieve symptoms of rheumatoid arthritis.

If, however, you do not feel dairy foods are a problem for you, then moderate amounts of no- and low-fat dairy products can be one good source of calcium. Many nondairy "milks" and cheeses made from soy, rice, or nuts, however, are also available on the market, and fortified versions provide a good source of calcium as well.

Gluten and Yeast

We group these two ingredients together because they often appear together in breads, cakes, and other baked goods. Gluten is a special type of protein that is found in wheat, rye, and many other grains. Approximately 15 percent of the population in the United States has gluten sensitivity in some form, including celiac disease and mild gluten intolerance, and many people with fibromyalgia are sensitive to gluten to some degree. Although both celiac disease and gluten intolerance involve a reaction to gluten, they are not the same condition. Celiac disease is an immune system reaction that involves a severe sudden allergic response to gluten. It is also characterized by malabsorption of nutrients, which can ultimately lead to malnutrition if not treated with the proper diet.

Gluten intolerance usually has a slower onset than celiac disease and can be difficult to diagnose because it can have a wide range of symptoms. Both celiac disease and gluten intolerance can be exacerbated by stress, infection, surgery, and pregnancy. Symptoms of both conditions can include weight loss or weight gain, constipation, diarrhea, gas, pain bloating, aching joints, depression, eczema, headaches, fatigue, irritability, cramps, and tingling and numbness. Although the evidence is largely anecdotal, people with fibromyalgia who eliminate gluten products from their diet frequently experience an improvement in symptoms.

In the case of yeast, some experts say it promotes the overgrowth of the yeast fungus in the body. This overgrowth may cause or stimulate joint and muscle pain. Eliminating foods that contain yeast may bring you some relief as well.

Monosodium Glutamate

Better known as MSG, this additive and flavor enhancer is found in a great number of processed and frozen foods. Like aspartame, it is an excitotoxin and so has the same ability to stimulate NMDA receptors. MSG often "hides" in foods under aliases, including glutamate, sodium caseinate, hydrolyzed vegetable protein, texturized protein, natural flavoring, yeast extract, and many others. Also, results of a 2007 study suggested that increases in glutamate in muscles may contribute to pain sensitivity.

Nightshade Vegetables

This is a difficult call to make, because the nightshade vegetables, which include tomatoes, potatoes, eggplant, and chili and bell peppers, are good sources of nutrients. However, in some people, there is evidence that consuming these vegetables triggers flare-ups of various types of arthritis, including fibromyalgia and rheumatoid arthritis. The exact reason for this reaction is not clearly understood, although some experts believe the vegetables contain substances that act as neurotoxins, which can trigger pain.

Eliminating nightshade vegetables from your diet is worth trying. If you do not see a change after a few weeks, then you can add these nutritious foods back into your diet.

Nitrates

Nitrates are preservatives commonly used in processed meats like bologna, bacon, deli meats, hot dogs, and sausage. Nitrates have been banned from baby foods because they have a toxic effect: they affect the hemoglobin in the cells, resulting in less oxygen in the blood. Some adults, including those who do not have fibromyalgia, experience symptoms if they eat foods that contain nitrates, such as difficulty breathing, dizziness, headaches, nausea, and vomiting. People with fibromyalgia can experience intensified symptoms, including pain, if they eat foods containing this preservative. So it may be best to avoid these foods. If you are "hooked" on these processed meats, try the vegetarian versions—they do not contain nitrates!

Phosphates/Phosphoric Acid

Phosphates are preservatives that prevent chemical changes of food that influence texture, flavor, color, and appearance. These additives also attract trace minerals in foods and remove them from the body, which can result in dietary deficiencies that could contribute to osteoporosis. Anything that promotes nutritional deficiency in people who have fibromyalgia needs to be avoided as much as possible. Phosphates in the form of phosphoric acid acidify and flavor cola beverages. Calcium and ammonium phosphates serve as food for yeast in baking, and sodium aluminum phosphate is a leavening agent in baking. Phosphates and phosphoric acid are found in baked goods, cheese, powdered foods, cured meat, soft drinks, breakfast cereals, and dehydrated potatoes.

Sugar and Simple Carbohydrates

Reducing your consumption of sugar and simple carbohydrates is good nutritional sense, but there is another reason related to fibromyalgia: sugar feeds yeast infections, and these infections are common among people with fibromyalgia. Another reason to cut out the sweet stuff is that when these foods are cut from a person's diet, weight loss often results, and that can help with fibromyalgia symptoms as well.

Another effect from eating sugary foods, including those that contain fructose and high fructose corn syrup, is the sudden spike in blood sugar levels, which is followed by a "fall" that can worsen the fatigue a person with fibromyalgia experiences. The "sugar low" creates more cravings for sugar, which is then followed by more fatigue, and the person is caught in a vicious cycle. Cutting out sugar and reducing

DID YOU KNOW?

If you have irritable bowel syndrome, you may feel much better if you avoid the following foods: fats, fructose, milk products, chocolate, alcohol, caffeine, and carbonated soft drinks. These foods can cause cramping, gas, diarrhea, bloating, and constipation. Focus instead on a whole-food, high-fiber diet.

intake of other simple carbohydrates can help fibromyalgia patients better control their blood sugar levels, improve fatigue, and perhaps even get some pain relief.

A VEGETARIAN OR RAW FOODS DIET

Only a few small studies have been done to investigate whether following a vegetarian or raw foods diet can improve symptoms of fibromyalgia, and the results have been encouraging. One study involved only 10 patients, who reported an improvement in well-being after following a vegetarian diet for three weeks.

In another study, all the participants adopted a raw foods approach for three months. The investigators saw significant improvement in pain, including substantially less morning stiffness. However, even though they felt better when eating raw foods, none of the subjects chose to continue with the raw foods lifestyle once the trial was over, and any benefits they had enjoyed disappeared once they returned to their regular diet. While it is understandable that a raw foods diet is a dramatic change for most people, the researchers noted that the fact that the patients' symptoms returned to their pre-study level clearly showed the association between diet and fibromyalgia.

In a study published in *BMC Complementary and Alternative Medicine* in 2001, researchers studied how a vegetarian diet would affect a group of 18 people who had fibromyalgia. For seven months the participants were instructed to follow a diet that consisted of fresh fruits, salads, raw vegetables, nuts, seeds, whole-grain foods tubers, flaxseed oil, extra virgin olive oil and carrot juice. They were asked to avoid alcohol, caffeine, anything that contained refined sugar corn syrup, refined and/or hydrogenated oil, refined flour, dairy, eggs, and all meat. They also included dehydrated barley grass juice powder as part of their diet.

Overall, the participants consumed more fruits and vegetables and thus more fiber, vitamin C, folate, beta-carotene, vitamin E, potassium, and magnesium than the average American does, and they also ate only small amounts of animal products, especially meat, poultry, and fish. Along with the dietary changes came an improvement in the patients' symptoms, but because the intake of so many different nutrients had improved, the researchers could not say which one, or ones, might be responsible for the patients' feeling better. They concluded that the improvement was, like the syndrome itself, the synergistic result of several factors.

Researchers compared a raw foods, vegan diet against the standard American diet in 33 people with fibromyalgia. Eighteen participants followed the vegan path while the remaining 15 ate as they normally did. Over the three-month period of the study, those in the vegan diet group experienced a significant improvement in pain, joint stiffness, and quality of sleep. Most of the participants were overweight at the beginning of the study, and those who shifted to vegan food had a significant reduction in body mass index along with a drop in their cholesterol levels.

A FEW WORDS ON WEIGHT

The dietary suggestions discussed in this chapter are good not only for helping deal with fibromyalgia symptoms, but also can assist with weight loss. A new large study published in May 2010 in *Arthritis Care and Research* found that being overweight significantly increases a woman's risk of developing fibromyalgia. Carrying excess weight also places a great deal of stress on the joints, which contributes to pain, and can make it more difficult (or make you feel less like wanting) to exercise. Thus, the relationship between following a nutritious, whole-food diet and weight loss is a winning one, and one we hope you will pursue. If you need help developing a weight loss plan, talk to a nutritionist, dietitian, or your physician.

DO YOU NEED NUTRITIONAL SUPPLEMENTS?

Living with a chronic condition places a great deal of stress on your body, which can cause you to lose vital nutrients. Even if you follow a varied, nutritious diet as much as possible, you may want to take one or more nutritional supplements. We did discuss several nutritional supplements in Chapter 8 that can be beneficial, including the ACES (vitamins A, C, and E plus selenium), B-complex, magnesium, and omega-3 fatty acids. However, before you choose a nutritional supplement, consult your healthcare provider or a certified nutritionist who can review your diet, state of health, any medications and other supplements you may be taking, and the reasons why you want to take a supplement.

THE BOTTOM LINE

The best fibromyalgia diet for you is the one that you create for yourself that not only meets your unique needs and food preferences, but one that is most of all well-balanced and based on natural, whole foods, and does not exacerbate your symptoms. If you are overweight, following such a diet, with the help of a knowledgeable professional, can also help you achieve and maintain a healthy weight. To establish that diet will likely be a process of trial and error. You may need to develop a food journal to help you with the creation of your own special dietary needs, and that is just one of the suggestions we discuss in the chapter on support systems.

CHAPTER TEN

Making Healthy Lifestyle Choices

Having fibromyalgia changes your life. If you used to be spontaneous, ready to try anything with little notice, now you likely feel as though those days are long gone. If you used to travel a lot, now getting out of bed and going into the kitchen can sometimes feel like a long journey. If once you enjoyed skiing, skating, dancing, tennis, or any number of other activities, you now find yourself delegated to the sidelines as a spectator.

But you don't have to be a spectator in life: although having fibromyalgia can change your life, you have choices, and when you exercise your options, you take back some of the power the syndrome can have over you.

In this chapter we explore some of the lifestyle changes you can make that can allow you to take back control of your life.

TRAVELING WITH FIBROMYALGIA

You want to be able to go on vacation with your family, leave town and visit friends, take a long weekend in the country. But you worry that your symptoms will flare up and that you will ruin not only your vacation but that of your family and friends as well. What can you do?

Although no one can guarantee that you won't have a sudden flare-up of symptoms the minute you hit the beach, you also must decide whether you want to be held captive by fibromyalgia or if you want to fight back. That's not to say that you should make the decision to go away on vacation or a trip without taking some precautions. However, if you do take steps to minimize the possibility of a flare-up and you are prepared ahead of time in case one occurs while you are away, then you will know that you made an informed decision and that it was the very best choice for you. Along with being cautions, it is equally important to try to live your life to the fullest extent possible. With that in mind, here are some tips that may help you enjoy a successful vacation with fibromyalgia.

- Get lots of rest before, during, and after your trip. A vacation or other type of travel requires a great deal of energy and planning.

  - **Think ahead.** To make sure you do not get overtired before you even leave on your trip, allow yourself to get extra rest for the few days before you leave. Do not pack all at once: think about what you want to pack, make a list, and then gradually add the items to your travel bags. Enlist the help of other family members or friends for packing or any of the planning that needs to be done before you leave. If you will be traveling with others, let them know ahead of time that you will not be joining them on all the activities, but that you will participate when you can.
  - **Pace yourself.** During the trip, take breaks throughout the day. If you are with other people and they have many activities planned, do not feel obligated to do all of them. Choose only those activities that you can do comfortably. You need time to rest and relax so you will have the energy to enjoy the activities you can do.
  - Once you return from your trip, allow yourself a few days to recover. Get extra rest, and do not

unpack right away unless you can have someone
else do it for you. Take your time.

• **Be a planner.** The amount of planning involved for
your trip depends on where you are going, if other
people are going with you, if there is a tour guide or
other travel help involved, what mode of transportation you are taking, and what you want to accomplish
on the trip. If you are going by car, you may need to
plan a certain number of stops along the way for breaks.
Whether you travel by car or plane, you may want to
bring along a travel pillow or other items that will
make you comfortable. Most of today's airlines (unless you are traveling overseas) do not provide pillows, blankets, or food. Plan to bring along a healthy
snack—don't count on airport food! You may also
need to plan ahead if you will need a wheelchair, a
motorized cart, or if you want to stay at a facility that
has certain amenities, such as a pool, whirlpool, or
massage therapy. Do you need a special diet? Check
ahead to make sure you can get the food you need. Do
you experience sleep problems? Although there is no
guarantee that you will get a comfortable bed, you can
call ahead and ask what kind of mattresses they use in
the hotel. Another detail is to plan each day's activities
ahead of time and write them down, so you know
what to expect each day. This does not mean you will
be participating in every activity, but it is good to see
what your options are in black and white.

• **Communicate your challenges.** If you are going on
your trip with your spouse or partner, other family
members, or friends, they should be made aware of
what your limitations may be. You need to communicate this before you leave on the trip so that there are
no misunderstandings or disappointments once you

are on vacation. This can be especially important for children, who may think mommy or daddy will be doing everything they have on their wish list. You are also doing yourself a favor by revealing everything before you leave, because you reduce the chance that you will try to do more than you should because you feel guilty or pressured into participating in activities you should avoid.

- **Be realistic about your expectations.** It is important that you think about your goals for the trip before you leave. This is a good time to write down your goals in your journal so you can look at them. The fact that you are making an informed, well-thought-out travel plan is a huge step. It can be a big emotional advantage to you if you view your vacation as an achievement just because you are going, and not for all the activities you think you can do while on the trip. If you look at your trip with these eyes, then you will not be disappointed if you do not accomplish all of your goals. Making the trip and being with your loved ones is accomplishment enough. What you learn from your first trip can serve you well when you plan your next one!

- **Keep up with your exercise.** Just because you are going on vacation does not mean you are also taking a vacation from your exercise program. At the very minimum, do your stretching exercises every day, especially on those days that you have to sit for an extended period of time.

CONTROLLING YOUR WEIGHT

Weight gain and obesity are significant problems among people who have fibromyalgia. Achieving and maintaining a healthy weight should be a priority, as recent research published in the April 2010 issue of *Rheumatology International* reports that weight control can be an effective tool in improving symptoms of the syndrome.

This makes sense. Extra weight places excess stress on the joints, the heart, and many other parts of the body. Carrying excess weight can make you more fatigued, less likely to want to exercise, and can contribute to feelings of depression. Overweight individuals are also more likely to suffer from sleep apnea, which can disturb sleep and leave you feeling fatigued all day.

In another study, published in the June 2010 issue of the *Journal of Pain*, the researchers conducted a study to look at the relationships between fibromyalgia and obesity and certain symptoms. In the study, 215 patients with fibromyalgia completed self-report inventories to evaluate symptoms, underwent tender point examination, participated in physical performance testing, and had a seven-day home sleep assessment. Nearly half of the patients were obese and another 30 percent were overweight.

The investigators found that obesity was related to significantly greater sensitivity to pain, reduced physical strength and lower-body flexibility, shorter time asleep, and greater restlessness during sleep. These results indicate that obesity may worsen symptoms of fibromyalgia and that weight management may need to be included as part of patients' treatment programs.

BEING A MOM WITH FIBROMYALGIA

Being a mom can be one of the most fulfilling "jobs" in the world, but it also demands a lot of physical, emotional, and mental energy. Fibromyalgia robs you of all of these in varying degrees, which means the world's hardest job just got harder.

If you have one or more children, dealing with your symptoms and raising a family can be too much for many mothers. Much depends on your situation—whether you have a spouse or partner who can help with the children, the age of the children, whether you have a job outside the home, of if other family members are able to help. In any case, being a mom who has fibromyalgia is a balancing act, and we would like to offer you some ideas on how to better juggle your responsibilities and take care of yourself at the same time.

- **Make a mommy signal light**. If you have young children, this simple tools can be a lifesaver. A mommy signal light can be posted in a prominent place—the door of the refrigerator is convenient—and this signal light system will let your family know, in a simple yet clear way, how you feel each day. Children as young as three years old can understand a simple color system. You can even enlist your children to help make the signal light. Draw or cut out of cardboard something that resembles a traffic signal light. Give it three "light" spots where you can put a different stick-on color: red, yellow, or green. The lights can be made out of construction paper or colored cardboard, which can be attached to the signal light with Velcro strips, or you may want to use red, yellow, and green magnets. In the morning when you get up, put the appropriate color into the spot on the signal light that indicates how you feel. Red is "I'm not up to going out today," yellow is "I'm operating at half speed," and green is "I'm feeling well enough to go out today." These are only suggestions: you can devise your own explanations of your coloring scheme. You can change your color throughout the day as your physical and/or mental status changes. Everyone will know at a glance how you feel and they don't have to keep asking you.

- **Go out with your children.** Meeting the demands of young children is tiring for people who don't have fibromyalgia, so it can be a monumental challenge for those who do. One way is to only take your children out on days when you feel well enough to do so: don't push yourself. (Hint: Use the mommy signal light to let your children know how you feel.) Before you leave the house, decide to do only the activities and errands that are essential. If possible, bring along another adult to help you. Pack an activity bag filled with your children's favorite books, toys, and travel games so they can be occupied while you are busy with errands.

- **Give up multitasking.** Have you ever heard the old Pennsylvania Dutch saying, "The hurrier I go, the behinder I get"? It seems the old wisdom was right. Studies show that a multitasking lifestyle may actually interfere with productivity rather than enhance it. A study from the Massachusetts Institute of Technology (MIT) found that people who multitask can suffer lasting neurological, physical, and social effects. You certainly don't need these complications! Therefore, prioritize and choose one task at a time that needs to get done. If you must take breaks, take them. When you complete that task, you will have a sense of accomplishment instead of frustration if you tried to start two or three tasks and were unable to finish any of them.

- **Assign chores.** This goes along with giving up multitasking. If you assign chores to your children (and spouse), you relieve yourself of worries about getting tasks accomplished, and your children can learn to understand that household tasks and responsibilities can be a family effort. It is also an opportunity for all of you to share time together. Perhaps have a treat (an easy one) ready at the end, such as making popcorn or watching a favorite video.

RAISING A CHILD WHO HAS FIBROMYALGIA

Approximately one in six people who has fibromyalgia syndrome is younger than 18 years old. As in adults, the majority of younger people with fibromyalgia are female. Young people experience most of the same symptoms that adults do, and treatment strategies are similar as well. The good news about fibromyalgia in children, however, is that the condition improves more rapidly than it does in adults, and in some cases children even outgrow the syndrome.

If your child has been diagnosed with fibromyalgia, there is a good chance that either you or your spouse/partner also has the syndrome. Therefore, you may be sharing the experience and the challenges together. Whether or not this is the situation in your case, here are some guidelines to help your child cope with his or her symptoms and treatment.

- **Communicate.** Speak to your child about fibromyalgia and educate him or her about the syndrome using age-appropriate language and materials. You can ask your healthcare provider for literature on fibromyalgia (materials for children if he or she has them available) so you can become fully informed about the syndrome and be better able to discuss it with your child. Certain Web sites associated with children's hospitals that handle fibromyalgia syndrome in children (e.g., Cincinnati Children's Hospital Medical Center; Comer Children's Hospital) can also provide you with information (see "Resources"). If you have a children's hospital in your area, contact them for information.

- **Inform your family.** Although you may not want to make your child's condition known to everyone in your extended family, it can be helpful to explain it to close relatives and friends, especially those who have frequent contact with your child. If these individuals are provided with accurate information, they will be better able to treat your child appropriately, and it can reduce any feelings of shame your child may have about having fibromyalgia. "I feel kinda weird having this disease," says twelve-year-old Rhiana. "But I don't like people reminding me that I have it. I just want to be like everyone else, even though I'm not. But my parents told my aunts and uncles and grandma, and they treat me okay, not like I'm sick." Feeling accepted is critical during childhood, and so informing your family members about the syndrome can go a long way toward helping your child feel better about him- or herself.

- **Join a support group.** Attending a support group with your child can help all of you better cope with the syndrome. A group that includes other children with fibromyalgia also lets your child know that he or she is not alone, and he or she can also learn new ways to deal with his or her symptoms from others in the group.

- **Make modifications to your child's schedule.** Many children who have fibromyalgia have type A personalities, and so these high achievers can become overstressed easily by taking on too many academic and extracurricular activities. Discuss your child's activities and stress levels with him or her and devise a plan that allows the child to keep the activities that are most enjoyable and eliminate those that are causing too much stress.

REVIVING YOUR SEX LIFE

"Sex life! What sex life?" That was the question posed by Rose at one of her support group gatherings. "I'm forty-one-years old and until I got fibromyalgia five years ago, I had a great sex life. I still feel like I want sex, but I'm always too tired and in pain. My husband has just about given up, and that frightens me. We are both way too young to stop having sex, but I don't know what to do."

Rose's situation is not unusual. Sexual challenges are common among people who have fibromyalgia. Some people experience a loss of sexual desire or have trouble with sexual performance. Others, like Rose, have the desire but their bodies don't cooperate. Muscle pain, joint stiffness, fatigue, symptoms of irritable bowel syndrome, depression—all of these challenges can keep you from enjoying sex the way you once did.

Engaging in sexual activity is healthy, and it can even help fight pain because it promotes natural painkillers called endorphins. A healthy sex life strengthens an intimate relationship and boosts mood. If you want to revive your sex life, there are some things you can do to help it happen.

- **Talk to your doctor.** Let him or her know your concerns and that you want to do something about it. If you do not feel comfortable addressing this issue with your doctor, there are still things you can do. However, it is best to let your healthcare provider know that you want to take steps to revive your sex life, because it may involve changing medications, which requires your doctor's participation.

- **Check your medications.** Some medications, especially the antidepressants called selective serotonin reuptake inhibitors (SSRIs) like Paxil and Zoloft, can reduce sex drive. Changing your prescription to another antidepressant or perhaps trying a natural antidepressant such as St. John's wort could make a positive different in your sex drive.

- **Try new positions.** There is more than one way to enjoy sexual intercourse, so it may be time for you and your partner to experiment with new positions that cause you less pain or discomfort. If you are a woman who has fibromyalgia and hip pain, you might use a pillow between your knees to stabilize your body during sexual intercourse. Pain in the lower back can be minimized by having intercourse while lying on your side. Paul, who has had fibromyalgia for three years, says he and his wife decided to try sexual intercourse in the one environment that was best for his pain: a swimming pool. "Fortunately we have a pool in the backyard, and sometimes at night, after our kid is in bed, we have sex. Before we discovered that this worked, we hadn't had sex for more than six months."

- **Be intimate without intercourse.** If there are times when even a new position you have discovered does not work for you, enjoy sexual intimacy without intercourse. You and your partner can explore ways to bring each other to orgasm without intercourse; try massage with scented oils (the partner gives the massage to the person with fibromyalgia and vice versa if possible); or get a book on sexual intimacy and discover new avenues of sexuality. This may be a time when you and your partner learn to enjoy each other in new, wonderful ways.

- **Go soak.** Moist heat, such as soaking in a warm bath or in a whirlpool, can ease fibromyalgia pain and may make it easier for you to enjoy sexual intercourse. Heat increases circulation and decreases muscle and joint stiffness. Other moist heat options include a moist heating pad, a warm shower, or a heated swimming pool.

- **Practice stress reduction.** Stress is known to trigger fibromyalgia symptoms, while learning how to control stress can boost your libido. Stress reduction approaches such as deep breathing, meditation, visualization, guided imagery, and yoga can release endorphins, which can reduce pain.

The bottom line is having fibromyalgia does not mean your sex life is over, but it can mean that it's time to make changes in how you enjoy sexual intimacy.

(RE)LEARNING HOW TO SLEEP

Establishing healthy, rejuvenating sleep habits can be a challenge and involves making some modifications to your lifestyle, but these changes are ones well worth facing. If you can at least partially tackle this symptom of fibromyalgia, you will be in a much better position to handle some of the others.

Some people who suffer with insomnia related to fibromyalgia seek help from a sleep clinic, but there are many things you can do on your own (or with the help of a few different practitioners) that could make your sleep problems better.

Here are some tips that have proved successful in various sleep clinics across the country. Information about the alternative therapies mentioned here are covered in more detail in Chapter 7. You should also consult your healthcare provider about your insomnia to determine whether there may be a medical reason (e.g., sleep apnea, restless legs syndrome, acid reflux) you are having sleep difficulties.

- Regular, daily exercise is likely to deepen sleep, while occasional exercise does not necessarily improve sleep the following night. Make sure you get your exercise at least several hours before you go to bed.

- Establish a regular time to go to bed and a time to get up, even when you have not slept much. Having a regular time to get up in the morning strengthens the circadian rhythm and leads to regular times of sleep onset.

- Avoid taking naps during the day. If you are extremely tired and need to take a nap, do not sleep for more than 30 minutes total. You may also restore some of your energy if you sit or lie down for 10 minutes without falling asleep.

- Make sure your sleep environment is comfortable. That means the mattress, sheets, pillows, coverings, and temperature need to be in your comfort zone. Because people with fibromyalgia are extra sensitive to pain and discomfort, even the wrong pillow may interfere with sleep.

- Your bed is for sleep, naps, and sex only. Do not watch television, read a book, work on your laptop, or anything else while in bed.

- Avoid caffeinated coffee or tea, chocolate, cola, and cigarettes. All of these are stimulants that can prevent you from going to sleep and staying asleep.

- Avoid alcohol. Although many people believe having an alcoholic drink before bed helps them sleep, the truth is that while it may help you go to sleep, it will wake you up once your body begins to metabolize the alcohol.

- Go to bed with a satisfied, not-too-full, not-too-empty stomach. A small portion of a high-protein food or a cup of soothing tea, such as chamomile, is good before going to bed. Avoid spicy, fatty, or heavy foods at dinner, as they can cause heartburn or gas and disrupt your sleep.

- Always go to the bathroom before bed. This can help prevent having to get up in the middle of the night.

- Avoid discussions or conversations that are upsetting before you go to sleep.

- Do something that will relax your body and mind before trying to go to sleep. You might listen to soothing music, practice relaxation exercises, pray, pet your dog, stretch, or meditate.

- If you do not fall asleep after 20 minutes, get up and do something relaxing. Avoid bright light while you are up because the light will have an impact on your circadian rhythm and cause you to feel more awake.

- Consider taking an herbal remedy that has been shown to induce a feeling of calm, such as melatonin, valerian, or chamomile.

If you have tried these sleep tips and you are still having difficulty with sleep, talk to your doctor. If you have been keeping a journal of all your sleep attempts, bring the information along with you on your visit.

DEALING WITH FIBROFOG

Symptoms of fibrofog can be one of the most disturbing features of fibromyalgia. Fibrofog, which is also referred to as dyscognition, is a state of mental confusion and memory loss that many people with fibromyalgia experience at some point during their illness. It can be aggravated by a wide range of factors, such as changes in the weather, excessive physical activity, physical inactivity, hormonal fluctuations, sleeplessness, anxiety, stress, depression, or mental fatigue.

"I thought I was losing my mind," says Mindy, a fifty-six-year-old real estate agent. "I finally had to take a leave of absence, because I couldn't concentrate on my work. When I began getting confused while showing clients homes, then I knew it was time to quit. I was really frightened until my doctor told me that fibrofog was common. That didn't help me with my job, but at least I wasn't afraid I was getting Alzheimer's."

Episodes of fibrofog can come and go; they may last for a few moments or stretch on for days. Once you are aware that you are experiencing fibrofog, you can learn to manage it. Here are some tips on how to alleviate some fibrofog problems.

- **Write things down.** Making notes for yourself accomplishes several things. One, it increases the chance that you will do the task on the note. Two, the physical act of making a note helps you imprint the thought more firmly in your mind. And three, it gets you in the habit of writing notes, which can make you feel less anxious about forgetting things.

- **Get treatment.** Many of the other symptoms associated with fibromyalgia—e.g., depression, insomnia, pain, fatigue—can make it more difficult to concentrate and remember things. Actively working to relieve these other symptoms can have a beneficial impact on fibrofog.

- **Stay physically and mentally active.** Regular physical exercise not only helps fight the pain of fibromyalgia, it can also increase your energy and clear your head. It is also important to keep mentally active by reading, doing puzzles, writing in your journal, and staying socially active.

- **Find ways to focus.** Placing excessive pressure on yourself or becoming anxious about symptoms of fibrofog will only make them worse. Instead, you can take steps to help you focus. For example, break up tasks into smaller steps, avoid distractions while performing a task, and avoid multitasking.

If fibrofog becomes a significant problem for a while, it may be wise to stop driving for safety reasons. Plan ahead and have alternative ways to handle any transportation needs during extreme episodes of fibrofog.

ON THE JOB WITH FIBROMYALGIA

Most people who have fibromyalgia continue to work after they get their diagnosis, but often the nature of how they work needs to undergo changes. Some employers do not understand fibromyalgia, so it may be up to you to educate them. While employees with fibromyalgia worry they may be laid off because of their health or because they may not be able to perform at the same level that they once did, employers are concerned about productivity as well, along with increased absenteeism, poor work quality, and the possibility of increased rates of work-related accidents.

Employees who live with fibromyalgia need to be their own advocates in the work environment. If you want to continue to work, and your symptoms are interfering with your productivity, concentration, or other aspects of your job, there are several people with whom you need to talk. If you work for a large company that has a health department or a health representative, speak with that individual about your experiences and your rights as an employee.

You will need to have a heart-to-heart discussion with your employer, and then with your coworkers. Because many people misunderstand what fibromyalgia is, you will need to educate them by talking about your symptoms of pain, fatigue, stiffness, and problems with concentration. Explain that you may have good days and bad days, but that you fully intend to make what adjustments are necessary to continue to be a productive employee. Offer to answer their questions. Your coworkers will appreciate your explaining fibromyalgia and that you are open about the syndrome and how it may affect your work.

Discuss with your employer some of the things you can do to maximize your productivity while also conserving your health and well-being. Here are a few suggestions:

- Ask if you can take rest breaks when you are having a bad day. You can discuss where you might take these breaks and how long they will be.

- Ask if you can take work home and complete it there if you are feeling too fatigued to continue at your job site.

- Ask if you can work at home on some days.

- Ask if you can take a nap during lunch break. It's been shown that a short nap is helpful for people with fibromyalgia and other chronic health conditions. In fact, people who suffer from insomnia could also benefit from a short 20-minute nap during the workday.

- Ask if you can come in on a Saturday or Sunday if you miss a day of work to make up for lost time.

- Discuss with Human Resources whether you can use sick leave for doctors' appointments and therapy appointments.

- If there are physical demands on your job that you find difficult or impossible to do, discuss this with your employer so a mutually agreeable solution can be found.

In addition, you can consider the following tips to help maximize your productivity and minimize your stress, fatigue, and pain.

- Utilize memory aids, such as schedulers or organizers, either on your computer or on paper—or both.

- Minimize distractions in your work area as much as possible. This may include correcting poor lighting (replace fluorescent lighting if possible and bring in a desk lamp), removing items on your desk or walls that are distracting, or turning off background music.

- Arrange your work area to be as physically comfortable as possible. You may need an ergonomic chair or need to rearrange your desk and filing cabinets.

FILING FOR DISABILITY

You want your life to be as it was before you were diagnosed with fibromyalgia, but you are experiencing changes over which you do not have enough control. Perhaps you are working full-time, but it has become such a struggle to fight the chronic pain and fatigue every step of the way that you ask your employer if you can work part-time.

DID YOU KNOW?

The controversial Irish singer Sinead O'Connor is among the celebrities who live with fibromyalgia. In 2003, O'Connor revealed in an interview in Dublin's *Hot Press* magazine that her diagnosis of fibromyalgia was a key reason why she decided to retire from music. O'Connor said that although she had a high pain threshold, she could not handle the fatigue.

Perhaps part-time work also becomes too stressful, so you decide you have to stop working. Your options? Because you are unable to work and maintain a reasonable level of productivity, you can apply for Social Security disability.

The Americans with Disabilities Act (ADA) has a general definition of what constitutes a disability, but it does not contain a list of specific medical conditions. Therefore, some people who have been diagnosed with fibromyalgia will be deemed to have a disability under the ADA while others will not. To improve your chances of being approved for disability, you need to do your homework.

There are laboratory tests and procedures for many medical conditions that can prove people have an ailment and thus they can qualify for Social Security disability. For people with chronic pain conditions, such as fibromyalgia, the proving part is more difficult. According to Social Security disability regulations, to qualify for disability payments you must prove that you have a severe impairment, an "inability to do any substantial gainful activity due to your medical or mental problem." If the Social Security department does not believe your claim meets this criteria, they will declare that you are not disabled.

To arrive at their decision, Social Security takes into account the combined effect of having multiple impairments, your age, and your education, as well as your remaining abilities and your work experience. You must be unable to do the work you did previously or any other substantial gainful activity. You will be asked for proof of your disability, including specific information about the trouble you have with daily activities, your limitations, and why you cannot work.

The Social Security Administration will ask for the names and addresses of your doctors, and each one will be contacted for your medical records. Your doctors should submit documentation of any prescription medications you are taking and any therapies and procedures you have undergone. You should be evaluated by a fibromyalgia specialist, usually a rheumatologist. If more detailed information is needed before a decision is made, the Social Security Administration may ask you to be examined by a doctor that they approve.

If you apply for Social Security disability and you are denied, do not be discouraged. It is common for fibromyalgia patients to be turned down on their first application. You can appeal before a judge who specializes in such cases. In some instances, it can be helpful to hire an attorney for the appeal process.

For more information about Social Security disability and how to file, visit the Social Security Web site (www.ssa.gov) or call your local Social Security office.

GETTING PREGNANT

Because fibromyalgia typically affects women at an early age, when many are thinking about starting a family, some women have questions about whether they should get pregnant and how pregnancy can affect their symptoms.

Every person who has fibromyalgia responds in a different way, so there are no hard set "rules" about what occurs during pregnancy. However, unlike women with rheumatoid arthritis, who often experience an improvement in their symptoms during pregnancy, women who have fibromyalgia typically have worsening symptoms, especially during the first three months of pregnancy.

Because pregnancy and delivery are high-stress circumstances, it is not surprising that fibromyalgia patients experience an increase in symptoms. Another factor that influences an exacerbation of symptoms is the large fluctuations in hormone levels that occur when women are pregnant.

If you have fibromyalgia and want to get pregnant, discuss your plans with your healthcare provider. You should make plans ahead of time to help reduce stress during and after your pregnancy. Some things that can help are taking regular rest periods two to three times daily, using moist heat twice daily, and exploring the possibility that you will need assistance at home at some point during your pregnancy.

You and your doctor will also need to discuss any medications you are now taking and what you should do while you are pregnant to treat your fibromyalgia symptoms. It is best to investigate alternative natural treatment options before you get pregnant so you will have a plan in place to replace the medications you are taking now. While herbal remedies may seem like a logical choice, remember that most herbs are not recommended during pregnancy because they have not been tested in pregnant women.

THE BOTTOM LINE

Having fibromyalgia changes how you approach and live each day. It forces you to take a new perspective on everyday routine activities, to come up with new ways to tackle old problems, and to approach new challenges with a different attitude. It can change your relationship with your loved ones, friends, and acquaintances, and the changes can be for the better. We hope you find that change is good for you as well.

CHAPTER ELEVEN

Finding Support

Living with the physical and psychological challenges of fibromyalgia is difficult enough, but for many people, there is the added issue of feeling isolated and misunderstood. Carolyn, a fifty-five-year-old former nursing assistant, says people have said to her, "Well, you look healthy!" when she has told them she has fibromyalgia. "What do they expect, a big red FM on my forehead for fibromyalgia?" she says. "I tell them, 'well, if you could see my insides, you would change your mind.'"

Fibromyalgia can severely impact every aspect of your life. When you have fibromyalgia, it can take all your physical, emotional, and spiritual strength to keep going, day after day. If you have a family, the responsibilities of maintaining a home and your relationships with your spouse or partner, children, and other family members can be stressful and even overwhelming. If you work outside the home, there are additional pressures you face every day. It is very easy to feel anxious and as if you have nowhere to turn for help and understanding.

Fortunately, there are support systems you can tap into in the community, on the Internet, and within your circle of family and friends. And yes, you can even draw strength and support from within yourself. The best time to reach out for that support is NOW.

COMMUNITY SUPPORT GROUPS

"What's nice about a community support group is that I don't feel like a freak. Everyone there understands how hard it is to get through the day sometimes. I don't have to explain myself or feel guilty about not being able to do something because I'm so fatigued." Brenda, a thirty-nine-year-old divorcee who works part-time as a graphic designer, attends a fibromyalgia support group at an area church once a month. She has made friends there, and they call each other frequently between meetings, sharing stories and offering each other tips on how to get by. Brenda says the group keeps her sane.

A support group offers a sense of belonging, of community. It is composed of different women and men who share a common problem, concern, or illness. A fibromyalgia support group can include people who have the syndrome as well as their friends and family members. In fact, participation by the loved ones of fibromyalgia patients are always welcome, because it helps them better understand the syndrome and how to build and maintain a good relationship with the patient.

Support groups can be large or small, be community-based or be part of a national or international organization. They can be held in churches, community centers, hospitals, clinics, or even members' homes. (There are also Internet support groups, which we discuss separately below.) Most cities and towns have fibromyalgia support groups, and the groups may focus on different issues, such as how to handle the emotional challenges of the syndrome or those that are centered on offering general information or how to survive in the workplace with the disease. Some people with fibromyalgia find that they like to attend more than one support group, including those that address related issues, such as chronic pain, chronic fatigue, depression, or irritable bowel syndrome.

If there are several fibromyalgia support groups in your area, you may want to visit each one to see what type of "program" they have. Some have guest speakers or offer field trips; some choose a topic to discuss at each meeting, such as nutrition, exercise, alternative forms of therapy, or medication use. Typically there is a lot of sharing of personal stories, ideas, thoughts, concerns, and tips.

Attending support groups can offer you invaluable benefits.

- You know you are not alone in your struggles. Even if no one else in your life understands what you go through, you know that there are others who share your feelings and challenges.

- You can pick up and share valuable information about others' experiences with different medications, therapies, healthcare providers, exercises, insurance issues, and diet. Because support groups are typically comprised of a number of different members and attract new people all the time, there is always new information available.

- You can feel a sense of hope. "Before I went to a support group, I felt so hopeless," says forty-eight-year-old Nadine. "My husband tries to be supportive, but my sister and my friends feel sorry for me, so then I feel sorry for me, and it's a vicious cycle. At group, people support each other, offer each other hope and encouragement. I need that a lot, and I get it every week."

- You can make new friends. Although you may have many friends who you have had for years, the friends you can make at a support group are special because they are part of your special world where you can be accepted for who you are.

Finding Support Groups

The National Fibromyalgia Association offers information on support groups (see "Resources"). You can also ask your healthcare provider or nurse and check with any local hospitals, as medical facilities sometimes serve as meeting places for support groups. Meetings may also be listed in local newspapers under "Activities" or "Support Groups," or you can search the Internet for fibromyalgia support groups in your area.

INTERNET SUPPORT

The age of cyberspace has given people with fibromyalgia and countless numbers of other health problems a new platform for getting support: Internet support groups, chat rooms, forums, e-mail exchanges, and the like. Internet support is at your fingertips, 24 hours a day, every day. If it is three in the morning and you can't sleep, your Internet support connection could be awake, too. Chances are pretty good that if you are awake in the middle of the night, someone in an on-line support group is up, too, somewhere else in the United States or anywhere in the world for that matter.

"The best thing about an Internet chat room is that I can find someone to talk to just about any time of the day or night," says Edie, a thirty-eight-year-old computer analyst. "I have made friends in several different countries and across the United States. We're all in different time zones, so I can always find someone who will listen or who needs me to listen. I live alone, so there's no one around to bounce things off, and my cyber friends are a great comfort."

Even if no one answers you immediately, you have the comfort of sending a message out to others in your group, addressing a question to a forum, and reading the latest chats and tips from other fibromyalgia patients who participate in these support entities as well. See "Resources" for online support groups as well as sites that provide articles and the latest news on fibromyalgia, information that you can access any time of the day or night.

KEEP A JOURNAL

One way to "take control" of a chronic condition is to keep a journal. It can be any type of journal that suits your needs: a symptom journal, a journal about your experiences and feelings about living with fibromyalgia, or a food journal that helps you keep track of the foods that do and do not exacerbate your symptoms. Or you could write one journal that includes all of these things. The important part is that a journal is **yours,** and you can choose to keep it private or share it with a significant other or close friend. You may even want to go to cyberspace and start a blog and share your experiences concerning fibromyalgia with others. It is up to you.

Keeping a journal is an excellent way to relieve chronic stress, allow you to get in touch with your emotions, and even discover new ways to live with the syndrome. Many people find that when they write down their feelings and goals, it gives those entities more substance. "At first I thought writing a journal wasn't such a great idea," says Lynda, a forty-year-old part-time bookkeeper and mother of a four-year-old.

"Someone in my support group was telling everyone how great it was to journal, so I decided to give it a try. Well, she was right. When I see my emotions down on paper, and I write down my goals, they become real. And when I accomplish them, I write that down, too, and it's a good feeling."

Getting Started

As always, the first step is the hardest one to take. Begin by getting some sort of notebook you can write in. Then make a commitment to write in your journal at least once a week and to include at least two items or topics each time. For example, you might document your fibromyalgia symptoms or feelings, things that triggered your symptoms, tasks you want to complete that week, a mini-goal that you set for yourself for the week, or any new foods that you tried and how you reacted. Once you have done this for a few weeks, you can increase your journal entries to at least three or four times a week.

Once you have established a habit of writing in your journal, you may begin to see a pattern in your thoughts and feelings about having fibromyalgia. If you write down things that trigger symptoms or when you have flare-ups, you can always go back and see if there is a pattern to these events. That's the beauty of having everything documented: it can help you identify patterns of events or things you may have done in the past that led to flare-ups. You can also go back and reread your entries to see if your feelings or attitudes have changed about having fibromyalgia and whether these, too, may have some impact on how you feel. In the end, keeping a journal could help you take better care of yourself and also make you feel as if you have some control over events.

Tips on Keeping a Journal

- Choose a type of notebook that allows you to be as creative as you want to be. If you are doodler, you may want an unlined journal. If keeping your writing in order is important to you, then a lined notebook may be better for you.

- Consider a scrapbook. If you like to keep mementos of activities or events, clippings from printed materials, or other things that are important to you, a scrapbook could be kept in addition to your notebook, or it could act as your journal.

- Choose a special, comfortable place where you can do your journal writing in private.

- Develop a habit of journal writing. Select a time of day and place every day or every few days, whatever schedule you find works best for you, and stick to it. It's too easy to say, "Oh, I'll get to it later." Later may never come.

- Make sure you date every entry.

- Your journal is private, even sacred, so keep it in a safe, secure place. Make sure other individuals in your household understand that your journal is off-limits.

- Writing in your journal should be a freeing experience, so do not worry about it looking or reading perfectly. Whatever you write will be perfect, because it is an extension of yourself and part of your self-discovery.

DID YOU KNOW?

It is easy to eat something without thinking about it or realizing it: you finish something on your child's plate, you taste food while cooking, a friend offers you something at her house, or there's a party at the office and you have a bite or two of something you normally don't eat. When you have fibromyalgia, however, those "forgotten" food moments can count a lot. If you keep a food journal, you are much more likely to become aware of your eating patterns and how they may be making your fibromyalgia symptoms worse.

FAMILY AND FRIENDS

Your family and friends know you have fibromyalgia, that you are fatigued and in pain and find it difficult to put one foot in front of the other too many days in the week. These are the people in your life who you love and who love and care about you. But love doesn't always mean they understand what it's like to be in your shoes.

Living with a chronic disease affects more than the patient; it can have a profound impact on the patient's spouse, partner, children, siblings, parents, friends, and coworkers. It is typically difficult for others to understand that while you look healthy on the outside, there is a battle raging within you, and you are fighting it every hour of every day.

That's why it's important to educate your family and friends about fibromyalgia.

You can do this in several ways. One is to ask your spouse, partner, or other close loved ones to accompany you to support group meetings. There they can hear about the experiences of others who have fibromyalgia and perhaps meet other family members and friends of fibromyalgia patients. Then your loved ones will know, like you do, the sense of community and sharing that can happen in support groups. Once they sense these things, they will be better able to understand what you live with every day. You might also share some literature about fibromyalgia with your family or attend an awareness event that may be sponsored by an organization such as the National Fibromyalgia Association.

Sometimes it is necessary to meet with a licensed mental health counselor or therapist to help everyone deal with the stress and misunderstanding about the syndrome. If you and your spouse or partner are struggling with issues surrounding fibromyalgia, couples counseling may help as well. If you have children who are having a difficult time understanding why their parent can't do things with them or go places when they want to, then separate counseling for the children may help resolve those issues. However, do not discount the power of going to support groups with your family. This is an option that you may want to try first because it is less structured and certainly less costly.

SEEK HELP FROM A THERAPIST

If people in the past have led you to believe that the pain and other symptoms you are experiencing have "all been in your head," perhaps the suggestion to see a therapist rubs you the wrong way. We are not suggesting you seek help from a therapist because we believe you are imagining your illness, but because anyone who lives with chronic pain also lives in a high state of stress, which in turn makes it more difficult to cope with everyday affairs. Therefore the suggestion to talk to a therapist is to help you learn how to better cope with living with a very real syndrome.

In Chapter 7, we talk about cognitive behavioral therapy, which is a therapeutic approach that has helped many people who have fibromyalgia. But there are other types of therapy that may benefit you as well. Theresa sought help from a spiritual leader, a woman pastor at her church who was also a psychologist. "She brought in a spiritual perspective that I really needed," says Theresa, a fifty-year-old office administrator. "I feel very comfortable talking with her, and I always feel uplifted after I leave her office."

Seeking guidance from a psychologist, psychiatrist, or therapist who deals with chronic pain or chronic illness can be very beneficial. Even if you attend only a few sessions or go once a month, you can come away with emotional tools to help you cope with the daily challenges of fibromyalgia.

THE BOTTOM LINE

No one should walk the path of chronic pain and fatigue alone, and there is no need to do so. Millions of people have fibromyalgia, and millions more loved ones and friends of fibromyalgia patients are out there, too, eager and willing to reach out, share, and help provide emotional, spiritual, and physical support.

SOURCE NOTES

CHAPTER 1. AN INTRODUCTION TO FIBROMYALGIA

Berenson A. Drug approved. Is disease real? The *New York Times* January 14, 2008

Buskila D. Genetics of chronic pain states. *Best Pract Res Clin Rheumatol* 2007 Jun; 21(3): 535-47

Buskila D et al. The genetics of fibromyalgia syndrome. *Pharmacogenomics* 2007 Jan; 8(1): 67-74

Guedj E et al. Clinical correlate of brain SPECT perfusion abnormalities in fibromyalgia. *J Nucl Med* 2008 Nov; 49(11): 1798-803

Lombardi VC et al. Detection of an infectious retrovirus, XMRV, in blood cells of patients with chronic fatigue syndrome. *Science* 2009 Oct 23; 326(5952): 585-59

Mork PJ et al. Association between physical exercise, body mass index, and risk of fibromyalgia: longitudinal data from the Norwegian Nord-Trondelag Health Study. *Arthritis Care Res (Hoboken)* 2010 May; 62(5): 611-17

CHAPTER 2. SIGNS AND SYMPTOMS

Lange M, Petermann F. Influence of depression on fibromyalgia: a systematic review. *Schmerz* 2010 Jul 4

Weil, Andrew. http://www.drweil.com/drw/u/ART00701/fibromyalgia

CHAPTER 4. GETTING A DIAGNOSIS

Celebrities with fibromyalgia: http://www.thirdage.com/fibromyalgia/celebrities-with-fibromyalgia/frances-winfield-bremer#ixzz0ssLSWzZJ

Staud R. Are patients with systemic lupus erythematosus at increased risk for fibromyalgia? *Curr Rheumatol Rep* 2006 Dec; 8(6): 430-35

Vargas A et al. Sphygmomanometry-evoked allodynia—a simple bedside test indicative of fibromyalgia: a multicenter developmental study. *J Clin Rheumatol* 2006 Dec; 12(6): 272-74

CHAPTER 5. TREATING FIBROMYALGIA WITH MEDICATIONS

Shaver JL et al. Self-reported medication and herb/supplement use by women with and without fibromyalgia. *J Womens Health (Larchmt)* 2009 May; 18(5): 709-16

Staud R. Pharmacological treatment of fibromyalgia syndrome: new developments. *Drugs* 2010; 70(1): 1-14

Arnold LM et al. Gabapentin in the treatment of fibromyalgia: a randomized, double-blind, placebo-controlled, multicenter trial. *Arthritis Rheum* 2007 Apr; 56(4): 1336-44

Holman AJ, Myers RR. A randomized, double-blind, placebo-controlled trial of pramipexole, a dopamine agonist, in patients with fibromyalgia receiving concomitant medications. *Arthritis Rheum* 2005 Aug; 52(8): 2495-505

Tofferi JK et al. Treatment of fibromyalgia with cyclobenzaprine: a meta-analysis. *Arthritis Rheum* 2004 Feb 15; 51(1): 9-13

Wood PB et al. Open trial of pindolol in the treatment of fibromyalgia. *Ann Pharmacother* 2005 Nov; 39(11): 1812-16

CHAPTER 6. EXERCISE AND MOVEMENT THERAPIES

Altan L et al. Effect of pilates training on people with fibromyalgia syndrome: a pilot study. *Arch Phys Med Rehabil* 2009 Dec; 90(12): 1983-88

CHAPTER 7. ALTERNATIVE MIND/BODY THERAPIES

Babu AS et al. Management of patients with fibromyalgia using biofeedback: a randomized control trial. *Indian J Med Sci* 2007 Aug; 61(8): 455-61

Baranowsky J et al. Qualitative systemic review of randomized controlled trials on complementary and alternative medicine treatments in fibromyalgia. *Rheumatol Int* 2009 Nov; 30(1): 1-21

Cuadros J, Vargas M. A new mind-body approach for a total healing of fibromyalgia: a case report. *Am J Clin Hypn* 2009 Jul; 52(1): 3-12

Gur A et al. Efficacy of low power laser therapy in fibromyalgia: a single-blind, placebo-controlled trial. *Lasers Med Sci* 2002; 17(1): 57-61

Hadhazy VA et al. Mind-body therapies for the treatment of fibromyalgia. A systematic review. *J Rheumatol* 2000 Dec; 28(12): 2911-18

Hsu MC et al. Sustained pain reduction through affective self-awareness in fibromyalgia: a randomized controlled trial. *J Gen Int Med* 2010 Jun 8; DOI:10.1007/s11606-010-1418-6

Kalichman L. Massage therapy for fibromyalgia symptoms. *Rheumatol Int* 2010 Jul; 39(9): 1151-57

Kayiran S et al. Neurofeedback in fibromyalgia syndrome. *Agri* 2007 Jul; 19(3): 47-53

Kroner-Herwig B. Chronic pain syndromes and their treatment by psychological interventions. *Curr Opin Psychiatry* 2009 Mar; 22(2): 200-4

Lush E et al. Mindfulness meditation for symptom reduction in fibromyalgia: psychophysiological correlates. *J Clin Psychol Med Settings* 2009 Jun; 16(2): 200-7

Martin DP, Sletten CD. Improvement in fibromyalgia symptoms with acupuncture: results of a randomized controlled trial. *Mayo Clin Proc* 2006 Jun; 81(6): 749-57

Mueller HH et al. Treatment of fibromyalgia incorporating EEG-driven stimulation: a clinical outcomes study. *J Clin Psychol* 2001 Jul; 57(7): 933-52

Schneider M et al. Chiropractic management of fibromyalgia syndrome: a systematic review of the literature. *J Manipulative Physiol Ther* 2009 Jan; 32(1): 25-40

Thieme K, Gracely RH. Are psychological treatments effective for fibromyalgia pain? *Curr Rheumatol Rep* 2009 Dec; 11(6): 443-50

van Koulil S et al. Tailored cognitive-behavioral therapy and exercise training for high-risk patients with fibromyalgia. *Arthritis Care Res (Hoboken)* 2010 Jun 2

CHAPTER 8. HERBAL REMEDIES AND NUTRITIONAL SUPPLEMENTS

Birdsall TC. 5-hydroxytryptophan: a clinically-effective serotonin precursor. *Altern Med Rev* 1998 Aug; 3(4): 271-80

Black CD et al. Ginger (Zingiber officinale) reduces muscle pain caused by eccentric exercise. *J Pain* 2010 Apr 23

Blecharz-Klin K et al. Pharmacological and biochemical effects of Ginkgo biloba extract on learning, memory consolidation and motor activity in old rats. *Acta Neurobiol Exp* 2009; 69(2): 217-31

Bundy R et al. Turmeric extract may improve irritable bowel syndrome symptomology in otherwise healthy adults: a pilot study. *J Altern Complement Med* 2004 Dec; 10(6): 1015-18

Cordero MD et al. Low levels of serotonin in serum correlates with severity of fibromyalgia. *Med Clin (Barc)* 2010 Jun 28

Forsyth LM et al. Therapeutic effects of oral NADH on the symptoms of patients with chronic fatigue syndrome. *Ann Allergy Asthma Immunol* 1999 Feb; 82(2): 185-91

Funk JL et al. Comparative effects of two gingerol-containing Zingiber officinale extracts on experimental rheumatoid arthritis. *J Nat Prod* 2009 Mar 27; 72(3): 403-7

Jurenka JS. Anti-inflammatory properties of curcumin, a major constituent of Curcuma longa: a review of preclinical and clinical research. *Altern Med Rev* 2009 Jun; 14(2): 141-53

Klein G et al. Efficacy and tolerance of an oral enzyme combination in painful osteoarthritis of the hip. A double-blind, randomized study comparing oral enzymes with non-steroidal anti-inflammatory drugs. *Clin Exp Rheumatol* 2006 Jan-Feb; 24(1): 25-30

Lister RE. An open, pilot study to evaluate the potential benefits of coenzyme Q10 combined with Ginkgo biloba extract in fibromyalgia syndrome. *J Int Med Res* 2002 Mar-Apr; 30(2): 195-99

McBeth J et al. Musculoskeletal pain is associated with very low levels of vitamin D in men: results from the European Male Ageing Study. *Ann Rheum Dis* 2010 May 24

Papakostas GI. Evidence for S-adenosyl-L-methionine (SAM-e) for the treatment of major depressive disorder. *J Clin Psychiatry* 2009; 70 Suppl 5: 18-22

Sengupta K et al. A double-blind, randomized, placebo-controlled study of the efficacy and safety of 5-Loxin for treatment of osteoarthritis of the knee. *Arthritis Res Ther* 2008; 10(4): R85

Shaver JL et al. Self-reported medication and herb/supplement use by women with and without fibromyalgia. *J Womens Health (Larchmt)* 2009 May; 18(5): 709-16

Shell W et al. A randomized, placebo-controlled trial of an amino acid preparation on timing and quality of sleep. *Am J Ther* 2010 Mar-Apr; 17(2): 133-39

Snitz BE et al. Ginkgo biloba for preventing cognitive decline in older adults: a randomized trial. *JAMA* 2009 Dec 23; 302(24): 2663-70

Turner MK et al. Prevalence and clinical correlates of vitamin D inadequacy among patients with chronic pain. *Pain Med* 2008 Nov; 9(8): 979-84

Valerian. University of Maryland Medical Center. http://www.umm.edu/altmed/articles/valerian-000279.htm

Warnock M et al. Effectiveness and safety of Devil's Claw tablets in patients with general rheumatic disorders. *Phytother Res* 2007 Dec; 21(12): 1228-33

CHAPTER 9. FIGHTING FIBROMYALGIA WITH DIET

Arranz LI et al. Fibromyalgia and nutrition, what do we know? *Rheumatol Int* 2010 Apr 1

Azad KA et al. Vegetarian diet in the treatment of fibromyalgia. *Bangladesh Med Res Counc Bull* 2000 Aug; 26(2): 41-47

Badsha H et al. Myalgias or non-specific muscle pain in Arab or Indo-Pakistani patients may indicate vitamin D deficiency. *Clin Rheumatol* 2009 Aug; 28(8): 971-93

Bennett RM. A raw vegetarian diet for patients with fibromyalgia. *Curr Rheumatol Rep* 2002 Aug; 4(4): 284

Castrillon EE et al. Effect of a peripheral NMDA receptor antagonist on glutamate-evoked masseter muscle pain and mechanical sensitization in women. *J Orofac Pain* 2007 Summer; 21(3): 216-24

Donaldson MS et al. Fibromyalgia syndrome improved using a mostly raw vegetarian diet: an observational study. *BMC Complement Altern Med* 2001;p 1:7

Smith JD et al. Relief of fibromyalgia symptoms following discontinuation of dietary excitotoxins. *Ann Pharmacother* 2001 Jun; 35(6): 702-6

CHAPTER 10. MAKING HEALTHY LIFESTYLE CHOICES

Arranz LI et al. Fibromyalgia and nutrition, what do we know? *Rheumatol Int* 2010 Apr 1

Glass JM. Review of cognitive dysfunction in fibromyalgia: a convergence on working memory and attentional control impairments. *Rheum Dis Clin North Am* 2009 May; 35(2): 299-311

Lapowsky I. Stop the multitasking madness! *NY Daily News* August 13, 2009

Okifuji A et al. Relationship between fibromyalgia and obesity in pain, function, mood, and sleep. *J Pain* 2010 Jun 8

RESOURCES

ONLINE SUPPORT GROUPS/CHAT ROOMS

ProHealth

http://www.prohealth.com/fibromyalgia/index.cfm

A "patient-powered" Web site that boasts message boards, a chat room, support groups, lists of organizations, events, and an e-mail newsletter. The Web site stays up-to-date with the most current news on research and treatment and input from fibromyalgia experts.

Daily Strength

http://www.dailystrength.org/c/Fibromyalgia/support-group

This Web site support group promises to get answers to your questions quickly, and lets you chat with friends; research the latest treatments and news; and create a wellness journal.

MDJunction

http://www.mdjunction.com/fibromyalgia

A Web site support group that advertises itself as "a community of patients, family members, and friends dedicated to dealing with fibromyalgia, together."

ORGANIZATIONS

ABC of Yoga

http://www.abc-of-yoga.com/

Comprehensive Web site on all aspects of yoga

American Academy of Medical Acupuncture

http://www.medicalacupuncture.org/

Offers a database of medical acupuncturists

American Board of Hypnotherapy

http://www.abh-abnlp.com/

Offers consumer information and a list of certified hypnotherapists

American Botanical Council

http://www.herbalgram.org

Provides comprehensive information on herbs

American Chiropractic Association

http://www.acatoday.org/

Provides news on chiropractic care, list of practitioners

American Chronic Pain Association

http://www.theacpa.org/default.aspx

Offers information, videos, FAQs, support group information, latest news

American College of Rheumatology

http://www.rheumatology.org/

Organization that issues the criteria for fibromyalgia diagnosis

American Massage Therapy Association

http://www.amtamassage.org/

Provides a magazine, consumer information, research, and a list of practitioners

The Association for Applied Psychophysiology and Biofeedback, Inc.

http://www.aapb.org/

Information on biofeedback, news, and a list of practitioners

Balanced Body Pilates

http://www.pilates.com/BBAPP/V/index.html

Information, podcasts, and help finding a Pilates instructor

Biofeedback Certification International Alliance

http://www.bcia.org/

Provides information on both biofeedback and neurofeedback, a list of practitioners

Cincinnati Children's Hospital Medical Center

Juvenile Primary Fibromyalgia Syndrome

http://www.cincinnatichildrens.org/health/info/rheumatology/diagnose/jpfs.htm

Information on fibromyalgia in children

Comer Children's Hospital

The University of Chicago

http://www.uchicagokidshospital.org/online-library/content=P01716

Information on fibromyalgia in children

Consumer Lab

http://www.consumerlab.com

Provides independent test results on nutrition products

Dietary Supplements Labels Database

http://dietarysupplements.nlm.nih.gov/dietary

Provides information about the ingredients in more than 2,000 dietary supplements, so you can compare ingredients in different brands

EEG Spectrum International

http://www.eegspectrum.com/

Offers a list of neurofeedback practitioners

Frequency Specific Microcurrent

http://www.frequencyspecific.com/

Offers consumer information, FAQs, a forum, and a list of practitioners

Herb Research Foundation

http://www.herbs.org/

Provides science-based information on benefits and safety of herbs

International Chiropractors Association

http://www.chiropractic.org/

Provides consumer information, list of practitioners, news items

International Institute of Reflexology

http://www.reflexology-usa.net/facts.htm

Provides information on reflexology

Light Therapy from the Mayo Clinic

http://www.mayoclinic.com/health/light-therapy/MY00195

Patient information on light therapy

National Association of Cognitive Behavioral Therapists

http://www.nacbt.org/

Provides list of practitioners

National Association of Myofascial Trigger Point Therapists

http://myofascialtherapy.org/

Provides some information and a directory of practitioners

National Board for Certified Clinical Hypnotherapists

http://www.natboard.com

Offers consumer information and a list of certified hypno-therapists

National Center for Complementary and Alternative Medicine

http://nccam.nih.gov/

Provides research-based information on alternative treatments for a variety of conditions

National Chronic Fatigue Syndrome and Fibromyalgia Association

http://www.ncfsfa.org/

Resources for patients and their families

National Fibromyalgia Association

http://www.fmaware.org/site/PageServer

Provides information on the syndrome and a fibromyalgia Support Group Directory to help you find support groups in your area

National Fibromyalgia Partnership, Inc.

http://www.fmpartnership.org/

Offers medically accurate information on the symptoms, diagnosis, treatment, and research of fibromyalgia, and more

National Institute of Arthritis and Musculoskeletal and Skin Diseases

http://www.niams.nih.gov/

Provides consumer information, research, news about clinical trials

Worldwide Aquatic Bodywork Association

http://www.waba.edu/

Information on how to locate a Watsu and other aquatic bodywork practitioners

World Tai Chi and Qigong Day

http://www.worldtaichiday.org/

Web site that offers comprehensive resources on tai chi and qigong

Yoga Alliance

http://www.yogaalliance.org/

Resources for people interested in learning more about yoga, plus a registry to help you find an instructor

FOR FURTHER READING

Arthritis Foundation. *Your Personal Guide to Living Well with Fibromyalgia.* Longstreet Press, 1997.

Balch J. *Prescription for Drug Alternatives: All-Natural Options for Better Health without the Side Effects.* Wiley, 2008.

Balch JF, Stengler M. *Prescription for Natural Cures.* Bottom Line, 2008.

Crotzer SL. *Yoga for Fibromyalgia: Move, Breathe and Relax to Improve Your Quality of Life.* Rodmell Press, 2008.

Davies C et al. *The Trigger Point Therapy Workbook: Your Self-Treatment Guide for Pain Relief.* 2nd ed. New Harbinger 2004.

Donoghue, PJ and Siegel ME. *Sick and Tired of Feeling Sick and Tired.* Norton, 2000, 1992.

Feldman, Christina. *Beginner's Guide to Buddhist Meditation: Practices for Mindful Living.* Rodmell Press, 2006.

Friedberg F. *Fibromyalgia & Chronic Fatigue Syndrome: 7 Proven Steps to Less Pain & More Energy*. New Harbinger Publications, 2006.

Hall MC. The *Fibromyalgia Controversy*. Prometheus Books, 2009.

Hulme JA. *Fibromyalgia: A Handbook for Self Care & Treatment*. Phoenix Publications, 2001.

Kunz B and K. *Complete Reflexology for Life*. DK Adult, 2009.

Lidell L et al. *The Book of Massage: The Complete Step-by-Step Guide to Eastern and Western Techniques*. Fireside, 2001.

Marek C. *The First Year: Fibromyalgia: An Essential Guide for the Newly Diagnosed*. Da Capo Press, 2003.

Mayo Clinic. *Mayo Clinic on Chronic Pain*. Mayo Clinic, 1999.

Rawlings D. *Food That Helps Win the Battle Against Fibromyalgia*. Fair Winds Press, 2008.

Schnellmann JG. *Understanding and Conquering Fibromyalgia*. CreateSpace, 2009.

Smith SA. *The Fibromyalgia Cookbook: More Than 140 Easy and Delicious Recipes to Fight Chronic Fatigue*. Cumberland House, 2010.

St. Amand, R. Paul. *What Your Doctor May Not Tell You About Fibromyalgia*. Warner Books, 2006.

Starlanyl, DJ. *The Fibromyalgia Advocate*. New Harbinger Publications, 1998.

Stewart K. *Pilates for Beginners*. Harper Paperbacks, 2001.

Williamson, ME. *Fibromyalgia: A Comprehensive Approach: What You Can Do About Chronic Pain and Fatigue*. New York: Walker & Co., 1996.

Wilke WS. *The Cleveland Clinic Guide to Fibromyalgia*. Kaplan Publishing, 2009.